CRITICAL A

"Cart this book along on your next trip (carry-on only, to be safe), and when things get bad, take heart from these veterans of the unexpected, unpleasant, and downright awful."

—*Trips*

"...the good doctor has our best interests at heart, giving expert advice, about learning how to eat and drink safely in a foreign country, including how to manage on long bus rides."

—*Las Vegas Sun*

"This one's concerned as much with what comes out as what goes in, and especially if you're doing the 'developing' world, it's worth digesting."

—*Arthur Frommer's Budget Travel*

"The book's strength lies in the very personal quotations of real people who aren't afraid to share their experiences."

—*Chicago Tribune*

"Such problems—and practical solutions—lie at the heart of this cheery and common-sensical guide to lavatorial hygiene away from home."

—*Independent on Sunday (UK)*

"We're a bit abashed to admit that this book, an evacuation manual of sorts, makes, um, a great bathroom read. The book gives straightforward advice and is geared primarily to Third World travel. But the best reading, if you're into potty humor, are the travelers' anecdotes."

—*Washington Post*

A SELECTION OF TRAVELERS' TALES BOOKS

Travel Literature
The Best Travel Writing, Soul of a Great Traveler, Deer Hunting in Paris, Fire Never Dies, Ghost Dance in Berlin, Guidebook Experiment, Kin to the Wind, Kite Strings of the Southern Cross, Last Trout in Venice, Marco Polo Didn't Go There, Rivers Ran East, Royal Road to Romance, A Sense of Place, Shopping for Buddhas, Soul of Place, Storm, Sword of Heaven, Take Me With You, Unbeaten Tracks in Japan, Way of Wanderlust, Wings, Coast to Coast, Mother Tongue, Baboons for Lunch, Strange Tales of World Travel, The Girl Who Said No, French Like Moi

Women's Travel
100 Places Every Woman Should Go, 100 Places in Italy Every Woman Should Go, 100 Places in France Every Woman Should Go, 100 Places in Greece Every Woman Should Go, 100 Places in the USA Every Woman Should Go, 100 Places in Cuba Every Woman Should Go, 50 Places in Rome, Florence, & Venice Every Woman Should Go, Best Women's Travel Writing, Gutsy Women, Mother's World, Safety and Security for Women Who Travel, Wild with Child, Woman's Asia, Woman's Europe, Woman's Path, Woman's World, Woman's World Again, Women in the Wild

Body & Soul
Food, How to Eat Around the World, A Mile in Her Boots, Pilgrimage, Road Within

Country and Regional Guides
30 Days in Italy, 30 Days in the South Pacific, America, Antarctica, Australia, Brazil, Central America, China, Cuba, France, Greece, India, Ireland, Italy, Japan, Mexico, Nepal, Spain, Thailand, Tibet, Turkey; Alaska, American Southwest, Grand Canyon, Hawai'i, Hong Kong, Middle East, Paris, Prague, Provence, San Francisco, South Pacific, Tuscany

Special Interest
Danger!, Gift of Birds, Gift of Rivers, Gift of Travel, How to Shit Around the World, Hyenas Laughed at Me, Leave the Lipstick, Take the Iguana, More Sand in My Bra, Mousejunkies!, Not So Funny When It Happened, Sand in My Bra, Testosterone Planet, There's No Toilet Paper on the Road Less Traveled, Thong Also Rises, What Color Is Your Jockstrap?, Wake Up and Smell the Shit, The World Is a Kitchen, Writing Away, China Option, Creative Spark, La Dolce Vita University

HOW to SHIT
Around the World

THE ART OF STAYING CLEAN
AND HEALTHY WHILE TRAVELING

TRAVELERS' TALES

HOW to SHIT
Around the World

THE ART OF STAYING CLEAN
AND HEALTHY WHILE TRAVELING

DR. JANE WILSON-HOWARTH

TRAVELERS' TALES
PALO ALTO

Travelers' Tales and Solas House are trademarks of Solas House, Inc.,
Palo Alto, California
travelerstales.com | solashouse.com

Portions of this book were previously published as *Shitting Pretty*.

Art Direction: Stefan Gutermuth
Interior Design: Kathryn Heflin and Susan Bailey
Cover Illustration: Amy Crehore
Page Layout: Howie Severson
Author Photo: Alex Howarth

Distributed by: Publishers Group West, 1700 Fourth Street, Berkeley,
California 94710.

Library of Congress Cataloging-in-Publication Data is available upon
request.

978-1-60952-192-9 (paperback)
978-1-60952-193-6 (ebook)

Second Edition
Printed in the United States
10 9 8 7 6 5 4 3 2 1

*By our bad habits we spoil our sacred river banks and
furnish excellent breeding grounds for flies. A small
spade is the means of salvation from a great nuisance.
Leaving night-soil, cleaning the nose, or spitting on the
road is a sin against God as well as humanity, and
betrays a sad want of consideration for others.
The man who does not cover his waste deserves a
heavy penalty even if he lives in a forest.*

— MOHANDAS K. GANDHI

AUTHOR'S NOTE

COVID-19 threw the world upside down in 2020. The pandemic killed, kept loved ones apart and scuppered travel plans but it has also showed our true colors, strengths and, perhaps, made us appreciate the value of family and friends and reminded us of the enduring rewards of travel. It has also made us aware of the importance of hand hygiene, respiratory etiquette and showed how bound to one another people are—wherever we live.

This new edition of *How to Shit Around the World* now looks to the future beyond the coronavirus. It focuses on the ailments that affect travelers and details the dangers of not following hygiene precautions herein described.

TABLE OF CONTENTS

This book is meant principally as a guide to avoiding illness and it is
not a substitute for a doctor's advice on your particular symptoms or
situation. If you are ill, it is always wise to seek a medical consultation if you can, and avoid self-prescribing if at all possible.

PREFACE

Fayre Cloacina, goddess of this playce
Dayli resorte of all ye human race
Graciouslie grant my offerings may flow
Nor rudelie swifte not obstinatlie slow.

—*Sir John Harington*

———

Living on the edge—that's what I feel like when I don't know what my bowels are going to do next. My eight-year-old son was more gung-ho. I could hear him shouting—from the Gents. We were in the fine medieval Castelo Lindoso in northeastern Portugal, and he'd rushed off to play Crusaders and Saracens with his elder brother. As I got closer, I realized he was yelling, "There's no paper!" The castle was close to the cottage we'd rented for a few days and, not realizing that the local microbes had made my son's bowel habits unpredictable, I hadn't put toilet paper in my pocket. There was none in the Ladies either so I shouted, "Use the bidet!"

"What's that?"

It transpired that there was a bidet in the Ladies but not the Gents; he was horrified at my suggestion that he come into the Ladies to get cleaned up, even though there was no one much around and continentals often use the Ladies if the Gents is busy and vice versa. The indignity of entering the Ladies was far more appalling than being "caught short" with a messy bowel movement. The poor lad was traumatized—for at least five minutes.

Travel is a joy, full of surprises and delightful new experiences. Perhaps some of the best times are those where one comes close to some disaster; the risks add spice, and make for great stories when you are safely back home again. But what are the risks of travel, and what is predictable? Wherever you are, you'll be eating daily and needing to go to the bathroom...but will you be able to identify the necessary "facilities"? And will the commonest of travelers' ills have you needing the bathroom rather too often? This little book will—I trust—allow you to enjoy your adventures with the minimum of forced gastrointestinal stops. Within these pages you will find strategies to avoid illness and ensure a healthy trip, if you wish. Because exotic eating is one of the delights of travel, I offer information to allow you to judge the risk of eating particular foods. You can decide whether you want to live conservatively or (relatively) dangerously.

The last time I was memorably ill with travelers' diarrhea was when I broke my own rules. I was out in the tourist quarter of Kathmandu. I didn't feel like waiting to eat in the busiest, most popular restaurants and picked one on the edge of Thamel. Inside, it was pretentiously decorated but deserted. Why was I going to eat in a deserted restaurant? Perhaps

I was fifteen, in the Casablanca airport with a full bladder. The toilets were obvious from their smell but the sign distinguishing Gents from Ladies was in Arabic. I entered the nearest to be confronted by indignant men using urinals. In my haste, I headed for the nearest cubicle. Once inside and my bladder empty, I realized what I'd done: I could hear the angry men outside shouting at me and dared not come out. Eventually a policeman escorted me to safety.

◆

Dr. Jocelyne Hughes, 38, lecturer in environmental conservation, University of Oxford, UK

there was a reason for its unpopularity. Would the food be stale?
I chose a Mexican meat dish, served on lettuce, garnished with
cold (probably unpasteurized)
sour cream and raw chopped
tomatoes. I awoke in the small
hours knowing I was about to be
very, very ill, and lay awake most
of the rest of the night waiting
for the vomiting to start. I
ignored my own advice, enjoyed
the meal, and paid for it, albeit
for a mere twenty-four hours.
However much you know about
avoiding travelers' diarrhea, you
may—out of adventurousness or
good manners—accept food you
would rather have avoided.

I have worked as a clinician
and health advisor in remote
regions for eleven years. On
many trips into inaccessible,
orthodox communities, I have
been treated as an honorary
man. I am offered delicacies. My

One of the curious questions I
am sometimes asked is what it is
like being a woman in a war
zone. Admittedly being the only
woman in the front line in a unit
of 2,000 men in the Gulf
brought one or two problems. I
could write a book for the British Army on the subject of
"Going to the Loo in Saudi Arabia," in a flat desert with no
bushes or trees. But in other less
exotic areas, such as Bosnia,
Chechnya, or Nagorno-Kara-
bakh, the question seems to
imply that there are no other
women in the region at all.

♦

*Kate Adie, OBE, BBC war
correspondent, Medicine Conflict
and Survival (1999)*

male hosts think that I am being paid a compliment, and the
celebrity treatment certainly facilitates my work. I am regarded
as having an intellect almost equaling a man yet I am allowed
to talk to their women even if they are kept in purdah. But the
biggest recurring problem I have in my honorary manhood is
finding an acceptable place to empty my bladder. One thing I
do early in any assignment is to find out how to ask to go to
the bathroom in a language most local women will

understand—and often this is not even the national language. My work took me to refugee camps in southern Bangladesh where I met many Muslims who had fled from the terror of the military regime in Myanmar.

What were the refugees' health concerns? One woman spoke for many: "When we first came, conditions were dreadful. There were no latrines, and we had to walk for miles before we could relieve ourselves without anyone seeing. Mostly we tried to wait and go at night. We got all sorts of bladder symptoms from hanging on too long, but now there are latrines, things are much better."

It is not only Western travelers who have problems finding somewhere to "go."

I've always thought that the British are especially tight-lipped about bodily functions, yet a lot of our humor is fecal, and we have some surprising

Mr. Johnson and I walked arm-in-arm up the high Street to my house in James's Court; it was a dusky night; I could not prevent his being assailed by the evening effluvia of Edinburgh…walking the streets of Edinburgh at night was pretty perilous and a good deal odiferous. The peril is much abated by the enforce [ment of] the city laws against throwing foul water from the windows, but…there being no covered sewers, the odour still continues.

◆

*James Boswell, Scottish
biographer of Samuel Johnson
writing in 1773*

place names. In East Anglia you'll find the village of Shellow Bowells (Essex), and further into the United Kingdom there is Wry Nose Bottom (say it out loud) in Cumbria, Crapstone (Cornwall), Shittington (Bedfordshire), Brokenwind in Aberdeenshire, as well as Shitterton and Piddle-in-the-Frome in Dorset.

Yet there is enormous scope for confusion and embarrassment when talking about the loo, even in your native tongue.

"My BMs are loose!" I could tell from her expression that this thin pale little girl was divulging some delicate confidence.

"What are BMs?" I hadn't a clue. Brits don't know that BMs are bowel movements, but when I *did* find out, how embarrassed we both were! She was a shy ten-year-old at summer camp in Connecticut and I was an ignorant, inhibited twenty-year-old Britisher not yet fluent in the local language. I was in a foreign country, without my parents and this was my first experience of discussing unmentionable things with strangers. Until then I had thought that only the English were truly obsessed with their bowels. Americans, it seemed, were interested, too, yet very coy, but there is an enormous vocabulary surrounding these embarrassing bodily functions.

How does one talk about one's bowel and bladder needs? How do you ask politely about

On a night train to Harare, I entered the toilet to find the light wasn't working. Returned to my seat, found my headlight, entered the toilet again, locked the door, went to sit down, and looked up into the eyes of a local holding the lightbulb. He was traveling without a ticket, hoping that he could hide in the dark undetected.

◆

Dr. Anne Denning, 37, ophthalmic surgeon, Bournemouth, UK

Closed the door of the windowless Parisian toilet. Pitch black inside. Felt for the light switch. There wasn't one. Came out. Looked for the switch outside. There wasn't one. Went back in. Still pitch-black. Still no switch. Getting desperate. Try anyway. Lock the door. Light goes on. Mon Dieu! Door lock is also the light switch!

◆

David White, 65, retired headmaster, Ayrshire, Scotland

the facilities? In Australia it's the "dunny" and each English public school has its own euphemism: at Winchester it's "the forakers," Lancing "the groves," Felstead "the shants," Leys "the Styx," Westminster "the japs," and at Malborough they go "to the woods." English vocabulary is rich. I might say that I'd like to visit the jakes; use the cloakroom; restroom; bathroom; lavatory; WC; privy; latrine; thunder box; john; karzi; bog; crapper; dike; roundhouse; the smallest room; the wee room; the necessary room; garderobe; the house where the emperor goes on foot; the honeypot; the thinking house; the throne room; powder my nose; pick a daisy; have a poo; be excused; spend a penny; have a Jimmy Riddle; shake the dew off the lily; wash my hands; view the plumbing; go and see a man about a dog (or a horse); take a dump; go to pinch off a loaf; got a bull in the chute; shake hands with an old friend; have a slash; splash my boots; go to the loo. Loo is said to come from the "*Gardez l'eau*" (Watch out for water) that medieval citizens cried before emptying their "pysse pottes" into the street from an upstairs window.

We haven't always been so coy; from the Middle Ages until the Victorian era, European royalty gave audiences in the garderobe, while the sovereign sat upon a "great stool of ease." Many Asians, too, are happy to talk explicitly. As a more experienced traveler, I was sitting through a long village health meeting in Lombok, Indonesia, and my bladder was getting fuller and fuller. Finally I had to ask. I leaned across to a female colleague and asked, "Where is the *kamar kecil* (small room)?"

"Do you need to throw away big water (have a shit) or small water (a wee)?"

I had been in the country some months but was still embarrassed by Indonesian directness. I didn't want to discuss my toilet needs, but when I said "Only small water," she took me to a bathing place with a minute drain hole in the corner of the concrete construction. I stood looking baffled.

"Just go there!" And she stood waiting and watching me.

"Umm…"

"Just go there!" she said pointing again.

In my embarrassment, my command of Indonesian left me, and I couldn't think how to say that I wanted to be alone. I weed hurriedly, pulled up my underwear, and fled, blushing. She stood there dumbfounded. "Don't you need to wash?" There: my filthy foreign habits were revealed.

The shared experiences within this book should help future travelers avoid humiliation when needing to bathe or use the lavatory. This book will also help reduce the amount of times readers will need to go to the bathroom: within these pages you will find the pearls of wisdom that will enable you to sidestep travelers' diarrhea, that oh-so-common of travelers' afflictions. So read on, and "go" in peace.

The Amazon city of Porto Velho has little space for the traveler seeking a quiet place to reflect. I rested weary legs in the small, dingy *en suite* bathroom of my budget hotel and sat on the toilet to read a few pages of my novel. Before long, a leaflet-bearing hand and then a face appeared through the door. The leaflet, in Portuguese, encouraged me to open my heart to God and let him into my life. The Lord does work in mysterious ways.

◆

Peter Hutchison, 32, author of the Bradt Guide to the Amazon, *London, UK*

INTRODUCTION
BY KATHLEEN MEYER
AUTHOR OF *HOW TO SHIT IN THE WOODS*

———

Travelers come in all shapes and sizes, lengths of hair and colors of fur and feathers. Those blessed with the DNA of humans, after surviving an escapade, will sometimes turn to writing about it. Thus, sweet as it is, the *raison d'être* for the publisher Travelers' Tales. In collecting and publishing the wild scrawlings of our stories, they also pass along—as with *How to Shit Around the World: The Art of Staying Clean and Healthy while Traveling*—hard-won, but invaluable, advice.

The yearning to explore the world and the genius for leisure wandering got their starts long, long ago, in all probability as outgrowths of survival-driven chases after migrating food and more hospitable climes. With the first crude dugout nosed into the water, the first sack slung over a shoulder, likenesses of you and me began evolving into a species of globetrotters, desirous—even more so than *Ursus*, the bear—of seeing the other side of the mountain. We've been known over the centuries for packing kit bags and departing familiar turf as hitchhikers, vagabonds, and stowaways. We sign up for overseas' jobs, we join the Peace Corps, we jet on our own time to aid victims of war, poverty, and natural disasters. Off we go to study—cultures prehistoric and modern, geology through its eons, a rare species of South African beetle. There are, of course, those of us content with walkabouts of more limited duration and extent, wanting nothing more than to traverse the river path, curl up under a tree, and dissolve into the pages of a good book. Then again, inspiration will chance along and spur us to build a raft and float it down the Mississippi, ride a horse across Cameroon, drive to Greenland, bag the peaks of McKinley and Everest, or retrace the high-seas voyages of Captain James Cook.

Whatever the occasion for our traipsing off to far-away places, within hours, we are all similarly confronted by the daily, away-from-home basics of eating, drinking, bathing, and excreting—and praying to remain sound as a bull doing so. Enter: Dr. Jane Wilson-Howarth, fellow of the Royal Society of Tropical Medicine and Hygiene, veteran traveler and revolving resident of countries from Nepal to Madagascar, Peru to Bangladesh. Prompted by a respect for diverse cultural customs and a longstanding fascination with parasites and intestinal pathogens, Dr. Jane offers up this guide to healthy sojourning. In it, she shares expertise derived from her ecological and medical backgrounds and her personal global experiences.

An Englishwoman by birth and heredity, Dr. Jane is not readily held back from thoughts about stinkers and squirters. From her scientific mucking about in the guano of many species, she is known to friends and colleagues as the Shit Doctor. I embrace her as a woman who can write with openness, intelligence, and humor on a topic that is still, in many circles, received only with titters and shame. Or, as Dr. Jane puts it, a certain, less-than-direct "coyness." Forthright with her advice, she may give some would-be travelers pause—in fact, pause enough to stay home. Yet others will be enticed to light out immediately—better equipped, as they will be—for far-flung adventures and mingling in non-industrialized cultures. Still, even the tourist playing it safe on a cruise ship, once schooled by Dr. Jane, may find that eating at an otherwise alien street stand becomes the high point of a vacation.

Expect to learn in the chapters that follow how to eat armadillo without contracting leprosy; how to avoid death-by-paralysis from things of the sea; and, somewhat indirectly—but not of least importance in a pinch—how to become a cannibal without getting Creutzfeldt-Jakob, the human form of "mad cow" disease. This last was of particular interest to me, being, as I am, a descendent of Scottish cannibals and continually going about in life never quite sure if, under duress, faint genetic leanings of this sort might just crop up. In addressing traveler's trots, Dr. Jane's emphasis on prevention is laced with instructive advice for those feeling that their lazily snaking twenty-seven feet of intestine has suddenly shrunk to a six-inch drainpipe. Rounding things out are tips on travel for seniors, people of special needs, and those accompanied by small children.

All the while we absorb the good doctor's treatments for our travel maladies, the pages of this book brim with their own "treatment" issuing from scores of travelers sharing their experiences in pithy, always entertaining, and often hilarious sidebars. Watch for the man in the wetsuit and the "chap" catching the train—my favorites. A bit of translation when it comes to the Doctor's British turns of phrase may be necessary for some of us: rest assured that "opening your bowels" does not require any type of field surgery, and the adamant promotion of "serious drinking" involves nothing beyond watery solutions of sugar and salt.

Once you light out, whatever little bit you haven't learned from Dr. Jane, you will discover for yourself, one way or another. Oddly enough, people along the way are frequently not only willing, I find, but eager, to toss open the ordinarily taboo topics of bodily functions.

So go. I mean, *travel*. Venture boldly out to loose yourself of the familiar and known; although, now and again, you may find yourself stepping in stuff, you'll also likely stumble right into the rich intimacy that, in so many ways, reifies us as a world family. For instance, the stranger who hiked up her billowing sari to demonstrate for Dr. Jane how to pee down a ceramic hole. Such straightforward exchanges pop up in the rarest places, resonate through the most curious connections, all told, serving as refreshing breezes, hopes replenished, in a more than screwy world.

Whatever you do, travel. Wherever you go, stay healthy.

Kathleen Meyer is the author of the international best-selling outdoor guide *How to Shit in the Woods: An Environmentally Sound Approach to a Lost Art*, now in its fourth edition, with more than three million copies in print, in eight languages. Her Montana memoir, *Barefoot Hearted: A Wild Life Among Wildlife,* was published in 2001. Meyer was the founding editor of *Headwaters,* the primary publication of the California organization Friends of the River, and has written articles for *Anvil* magazine, the *Professional Farrier,* and various Travelers' Tales anthologies. A lifelong outdoorswoman, Meyer lives in an old dairy barn in western Montana with her sweetie, farrier Patrick McCarron, one useless cat, a nursery colony of eighty big brown bats, and countless wild skunks, raccoons, marmots, and mice. Find her at www.kathleeninthewoods.net.

Chapter 1

TRAVELERS' DIARRHEA
KNOWING IT, AVOIDING IT

The young American put his head down to the milk-bowl and the
milk darkened, from white to grey, as his head blocked out the
light. The bowl was half a calabash. He held it in his palms and felt
the warmth coming through. There were black hairs floating on the
surface and a faint smell of pitch. He tilted the bowl till the froth
brushed against his moustache. "Shall I?" He paused before his lips
touched the milk. Then he tilted it again and gulped.

—*Bruce Chatwin, Anatomy of Restlessness*

———

Traveling is a little hazardous; that is what makes it exciting. But what are the risks? What about all those tropical diseases that are out to get you: plague, hantavirus, dengue, rabies, cholera, typhoid, typhus (what's the difference?), tuberculosis, dysentery, yellow fever, malaria? Malaria literally means bad air, the name originating from a time when the disease was rampant in Europe and people got it from venturing into dank, marshy places. No one understood how it was caught; it was a mysterious and feared infection. A lot of worries about this and other travelers' ills stem from misunderstanding or ignorance of avoidance strategies, but the following chapters explain how risks can be minimized.

It surprises many people that it is not tropical disease that takes most travelers' lives. It is accidents that are most likely to kill you. Infectious or communicable diseases take surprisingly few adventurers' lives: less than 4 percent of those few who do die abroad. Tropical infections don't kill many travelers, but that doesn't mean that we avoid illness: on the contrary, most of us get sick when we travel. The most common infection which gets us is diarrhea, and studies say that about half of those traveling to the low-income regions will get a dose of Montezuma's revenge each trip. The highest-risk destinations are tropical Latin America and the Indian subcontinent; North Americans import their diarrhea and dysentery from Mexico, Ecuador, Peru, and Bolivia, and Europeans bring theirs mostly from India and Nepal. It isn't just travelers who suffer either; the diarrheal diseases cause a lot of illness (and even deaths) in the local population, too. You only need to look at the consistency of the brown deposits on the streets of Kathmandu to realize this.

What is travelers' diarrhea? Diarrhea means loosening of the bowels so that the sufferer "goes"

> ——— ★ * ———
>
> Although we traveled for over a year in Latin America neither my husband nor I became ill with "the trots." We were not over-cautious about sampling local foods, but made sure we ate only food that was served piping hot. We ate street food, but only dishes that were cooked as we waited. We stuck to bottled water in most places.
>
> ◆
>
> *Karen Birch, 36, sales coordinator, Sussex, UK*

at least three times in twenty-four hours. The most common form makes you ill for around thirty-six hours then symptoms disappear without doing any real harm, except perhaps leaving a somewhat battleworn tail end. There are as many names for travelers' diarrhea as there are kinds of microbes that cause it. There is gastroenteritis, food poisoning, upset stomach, Montezuma's revenge (from Latin America), gyppy tummy (from Egypt), Delhi belly, the Kathmandu quickstep, Tandoori trots (from the subcontinent), the Aztec two-step, turista, the runs, the squits, the squirts, the screaming shits.... The most common culprit is snappily known as enterotoxigenic *Escherichia coli* or ETEC to those who know it more intimately. These little blighters produce a toxin that acts in the same way as cholera, stimulating an outpouring of water and salts into the bowel; the result is thirty-six to forty-eight hours of frequent trips to the lavatory to deposit said water and salts. Studies have shown that this is responsible for up to 40 percent of cases of travelers' diarrhea, and this is the most likely criminal especially in Africa and Central and South America. ETEC is the most common but there are others.

➤ Among ETEC's many cousins are: Enteroadherent, enterohemorrhagic E. coli, and others

➤ *Campylobacter*, causing spasmodic pains with the diarrhea

➤ *Shigella*, only ten bacteria need to get in for a brisk bout of bacillary dysentery (see page 59)

➤ Other bacterial causes of diarrhea, like *Salmonella* food poisoning

➤ *Giardia*, which will cause you to generate smelly emissions that will make you most unpopular (see page 60)

➤ A variety of other parasites and worms (see Chapter 12)

➤ Amebic dysentery (see page 59)

➤ *Cryptosporidium*, which causes a tedious type of diarrhea that lasts for two weeks with a lot of cramps; there is no specific treatment

➤ Rotaviruses or "small round viruses," aka Norovirus or Norwalk-like viruses and many others causing epidemic vomiting

➤ Cholera (see pages 63, 69)

➤ *Cyclospora* (see page 60)

➤ Tropical infections (like malaria) which can cause diarrhea along with other symptoms.

There is a range of nontropical, noninfectious causes of diarrhea that are unrelated to travel but may occur in travelers coincidentally. Just because you are traveling and you have diarrhea does not mean that you have travelers' diarrhea. See a doctor if in doubt.

The microbes that cause stomach problems abroad are many and varied, yet fortunately for us the prevention strategies and the treatments are similar for most of these. So where does it come from? Most "stomach upsets" in travelers come via a revolting route known by medics as fecal-oral transmission; I call it the filth-to-mouth route, or getting someone else's feces into your stomach. Someone has the Kathmandu quickstep and uses the longdrop lavatory but doesn't wash his hands before preparing your sandwich and soon you too are running to the loo. Most travelers' diarrhea gets you via contaminated food: food handled by someone with traces of feces on their hands. The term "diarrhea" includes the full range of filth-to-mouth infections listed above (the exotic ones are detailed in Chapter 8), but in addition there are filth-to-mouth

In the 1970s, Goa offered few tourist facilities. The toilet was a stone cubicle with two breeze blocks to keep the feet above ground level. The area between the blocks was puzzlingly clean. One day though, while I was squatting to empty my bowels, a small pig appeared and vacuumed up everything I'd produced. My dilemma was then whether to continue to tempt fate by eating those delicious local sausages.

◆

Jane Thakker, 46, sail-training coordinator, Warsash, Hampshire, UK

diseases (including typhoid, paratyphoid, hepatitis A and E, and some of the worm infestations), which cause symptoms other than diarrhea. All the microbes in this formidable list can be avoided by following similar, simple precautions.

None of these microbes survives cooking. However filthy the food was when it arrived in the kitchen and however unhygienic the chef has been, thoroughly cooked food will not harm you. Well-cooked, piping hot meals are safe, but food that is lukewarm or has been cooked, allowed to go cold, and then is handled by someone is risky. Cold dishes like quiche, pizza, and savory pies might be a source of Delhi belly if the food has been badly stored or touched with dirty hands. Meat is more risky than vegetarian dishes, because animals can become infected while they are still alive,

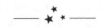

Bumped from our flight in Bogotá, my wife and I received a complimentary hotel room and a free dinner. Despite having horrible diarrhea, we, as a matter of principle, ordered the most expensive meal: shellfish and pasta. Over the next five hours we nearly divorced over access to the single toilet in our room. Toward 3:00 A.M. I discovered just how long the intestines are, as I noticed the parsley from my garlic spaghetti side dish in the toilet bowl. My attitude improved then, as I knew there was nothing left to come through.

♦

Calvin Dorion, 35, teacher, Cambridge, UK

and, once slaughtered, flesh is a better environment for the survival and multiplication of harmful microbes than is vegetable matter.

Salads are often grown in highly contaminated ground (people without toilets often relieve themselves in vegetable gardens), and low-growing fruits, especially strawberries, can easily become contaminated by human feces. The most hazardous raw foods are those that can trap filth in crevices and are difficult to clean—lettuce is among the worst. Conversely, smoothskinned items can be cleaned quite well, so carefully washed tomatoes and items that can be peeled like carrots or radishes are fairly safe. Washing or peeling is also advisable to reduce the amount of pesticides you swallow. There are no foods that are 100 percent safe, but the challenge is to reduce risks to a minimum, without making the traveling experience one of precautions, worries, and anxieties from morning until night.

There are innumerable myths about what causes bad stomachs in travelers, but it is nearly always contaminated food, or occasionally—just occasionally—dirty water. Mellor's *voice of experience* (this page) illustrates some of the common misconceptions of many travelers. The myth of

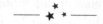

I drink the water provided by hotels abroad, eat on the street, and indulge in ice cream on a hot day. I believe that the introduction of a few foreign microbes into one's system assists acclimatization; if locals can eat ice cream without suffering dire consequences, so can I. I have suffered an attack of dysentery in India which rendered me fearful of relaxing clenched buttocks, and been laid low by a bug that debilitated me for the entire overland journey to Lhasa. Both were contracted in supposedly safe environments.

♦

T. Mellor, Middlesex, UK, Letter in Wanderlust *magazine (see author's comment below)*

locals being immune is ill-informed travelers' folklore, and the distressingly common idea that eating bad food will immunize you is responsible for a lot of unnecessary illness in travelers, as well as exposing them to dangerous filth-to-mouth infections like typhoid. In short, hot street food = safe. Hotel water = may be safe, could be chancy. Ice cream in India or Nepal = clench your buttocks.

𝒯*ips*

➤ Peel it, boil it, cook it, or forget it: this is the maxim to protect you from travelers' diarrhea and other fecal-oral diseases when visiting less sanitary places.

➤ In the Middle East and South Asia, some melon sellers puncture the fruits and soak them in roadside drains to make them weigh heavy before sale. This is a probable explanation of why, in the days of the British Raj, melons were blamed for Indian cholera outbreaks.

➤ Choose freshly cooked, piping hot food rather than reheated food or food kept lukewarm on a hotel buffet.

➤ Sizzling hot street food is likely to be safer than just-warm food, even if produced by an international hotel.

➤ In international hotels order à la carte foods if you can.

I was very proud of myself in Tyrona, Colombia; I achieved what most travelers could only dream of: painful constipation. The suffering was well worth the status amongst my peers.

◆

Calvin Dorion, 35, ex-pat Canadian teacher, Cambridge, UK

In a snack bar in Arusha, Tanzania, the deep-fried chicken was so hot that I had to hold it with paper serviettes. Yet as I ate, I discovered, too late, ice along the still frozen central bone. Driving along about twelve hours later, the salmonella hit me, and before I had a chance to pull over I emptied my stomach and bowel, and the evacuation continued in hospital for three days. Now I cut into my finger food and look at it before I eat.

◆

Steve Foreman, 47, explorer, Walesby, Nottinghamshire, UK

➤ In busy local restaurants eat what everyone else is eating; don't ask for dishes that are "exotic" for them.

➤ Avoid salads—especially lettuce—and also unclean- able soft fruits like strawber- ries unless these items have been grown and prepared hygienically. In Kathmandu, La Paz, and many other places, the only safe lettuce is boiled lettuce.

➤ Fresh mayonnaise can harbor *Salmonella* bacteria. These bacteria usually causes a week of severe diarrhea, with abdominal cramps and sometimes fever.

➤ Dishes containing meat are more likely to make you ill than vegetarian foods so becoming vegetarian when you travel will reduce stom- ach troubles.

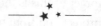

A market town in Hunan, China, boasted a hotel so grand that the latrines were indoors, on the second floor. Crouching over a drafty hole, I was alarmed to hear voices coming from beneath me. Imagine hearing voices coming from a lavatory bowl, you'll know how vulnera- ble I felt. I looked down. There in the room below was a thirty- foot-wide pool full of what came through the holes above; on the shores of this indescrib- able sea stood The Three Most Unfortunate Men in the World, ladling out fertilizer for the veggies. Salad is not a wise choice in China.

◆

Catherine Hopper, 37, cycling Buddhist, Manchester, UK

➤ Fried rice often makes people ill in Nepal, espe- cially if it is made with leftover meat. The ingredients have often been hanging around unrefrigerated and are often flash-fried and thus inadequately reheated.

➤ Pork and dog are the riskiest kinds of meat. Pigs and dogs are often the local rubbish disposal consultants where environmental hygiene is poor. Any pork (or dog) that you choose to eat must be very thoroughly cooked. Nepalis say that it is unwise to eat pork during the hot season—for good reason.

➤ In most non-industrialized countries, fresh milk—even milk that claims to be pasteurized—should be boiled before drinking.

➤ In Kyrgyzstan it is normal to put jam in tea, whereas you are expected to swallow fermented mares' milk straight. I'm not sure I'd risk it. Raw camels' milk too can be risky—it was found to be a source of the Middle East respiratory syndrome coronavirus.

➤ Yogurt is usually safe because the milk is boiled before fermentation and the final product is slightly acidic and thus less favorable for the survival of noxious bacteria.

➤ Sorbet tends to be acidic and, since acids are unfavorable to bacteria, this is a fairly safe food.

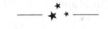

In Arambol, a one-tap fishing village in Goa, I came down with extremely bad diarrhea. Innumerable toilet visits had me teetering on two rocks sheltered by palm leaves; the balancing act was made more precarious by charging hungry pigs.

◆

Vincent Ward, 39, reluctant farmhand, Chiba-ken, Japan

➤ Ice cream is often risky in low-income countries since power cuts make it difficult to store safely, and it is microbe paradise.

➤ Ice, too, is often made with dirty water or handled with dirty hands. Sometimes it is delivered in huge blocks that are dumped onto the ground outside the drinks stall or hotel.

➤ The worst two meals of my life were cold old goat stew in Java and cold fatty lamb stew in Greece. Restaurateurs couldn't be persuaded to reheat them properly. They couldn't see the point.

➤ There are a few rare tropical infections that come via the filth-to-mouth route. These are hantavirus, which comes from eating foods that have been excreted upon or nibbled by mice; Weil's disease (leptospirosis), from swallowing food or drink contaminated with rat urine; and Lassa fever, which often comes from consuming food contaminated with the urine of the multimammate rat. Following two simple rules reduces the risk of acquiring all of these nasty but rare infections: eat your food piping hot, and drink safe water.

My worst experience of having the runs was when camping in Egypt. I woke up and found I had diarrhea everywhere—and I mean everywhere— in my sleeping bag. I could only clean up by going into the sea, and took my sleeping bag with me. There were no toilets I could use so I spent a couple of days right there on the beach.

◆

Shirley Thomas, 48, transcontinental cyclist, Leicester, UK

Chapter 2

WHAT'S IN THE WATER?
WHEN IS IT SAFE TO DRINK?

A POOEM

Hanging latrines can be fun
Everyone loves a shit in the sun.
Over fields, crops and lakes
We drop our curly little cakes.

And thus we spread so much disease
Without a thought, with consummate ease.
Worms, amoebae, parasites and cysts
Destined all for deadly trysts.

Spread by dogs, children and chickens
Provides–guaranteed–all that sickens.
Into our tummies they quickly go
For the rumbling diarrhea show.

So all tasty fruit please do peel,
Or your fate you will seal.
Eat nothing but hot cooked food
Then your health will stay fair rude.

—*Derrick Ikin, 53, poet laureate of the defecatorium, Maputo, Mozambique*

***

*M*ost travelers seem preoccupied with water quality, unaware that it is bad food hygiene that most often makes them sick. Perhaps one reason for this misapprehension is that there is a lot of investment in clean water and there is money to be made from selling water purification devices to travelers. There *are* outbreaks of waterborne illnesses—especially during times of civil unrest, war, tsunami, disaster, and chaos—but the vast majority of travelers' intestinal symptoms are due to poor food-handling practices. The reason is that contaminated hands can carry millions of harmful microbes, which can then be inoculated into food, breed to produce millions more microbes, and thus produce a very effective "infective dose" of harmful bacteria. Conversely, germs that enter clean-looking drinking water may die for want of food or may become so dispersed and diluted that when that slightly contaminated water is swallowed, only one or two bacteria enter the body and these are in insufficient numbers to cause illness. I am not suggesting that it is wise to drink any water anywhere, but that drinking pure water will not completely protect you.

Even in low-income countries the quality of domestic water is a lot better than it used to be, and many international hotels ensure that their water supply is clean. Ask if you are unsure. Studies in several Asian countries suggest that bottled mineral water produced locally may not be entirely safe. Most of it is not even "mineral water" but treated (or untreated) tap water. Yet there has been a boom in "mineral water" production so that it is available in a surprising number of quite remote destinations now. The quality is patchy, but if I need water in a city in resource-poor regions, I drink bottled water. It is usually safe enough. Other kinds of bottled drinks, the colas and other carbonated drinks, should be safe because the contents are

Corrie insisted that if the locals in Cairo could drink the water, so could she. She was hit with a severe case of the runs—the original "gyppy" tummy—and eventually sought medical advice. Despite treatment with vitamins and constipation pills in Egypt, she was still ill a month after returning home.

◆

Jo Surtees, 29,
wandering English teacher,
Iwate-Ken, Japan

somewhat acidic which is unfavorable for microbes, and boxed drinks will also be safe. Beware of "homemade" drinks that have involved a lot of handling during concoction.

If you need really safe water—you may be traveling with a young baby or your own health dictates that you must take special care—the safest means of treating water is to boil it. Water that has been brought to a good rolling boil is safe, and even water heated above 140°F/60°C is unlikely to harbor any nasty microbes. When I was traveling in the remote mountains of Nepal with my three-month-old, I carried a metal vacuum flask. Whenever we stopped to eat, or we stopped at a tea shop, I asked for the flask to be filled with boiling water. Kept hot like this for fifteen minutes or so, even water that has not been properly boiled will be ultrasafe. Another precaution:

I sterilize all drinking water with tincture of iodine. This is extremely cheap, and it is also widely available (from pharmacists), although you need to check the strength. I use five to ten drops per liter of the English variety, though rarely use more than six or seven unless the water is particularly suspect. I let it stand for twenty minutes before drinking. Although the bottle says for external use only, it is safe if used in this way, and has kept me healthy on many extended trips where pure water is hard to find. A vial of iodine is much lighter than a water filter (backpackers must consider weight). One drawback is the horrible taste, which I counteract with powdered drink: added in small quantities, it just takes the taste of the iodine away without making the water too sweet.

♦

Phil Brabbs, 42, teacher trainer, Plzeň, Czech Republic

very sensitive stomachs may protest if there is a lot of sediment in the water, and turbid water makes chemical sterilization methods less effective. Leave very turbid water to stand or filter it.

After boiling, the next best way of treating water is chemically. Chemical "sterilization" takes time (thirty minutes), gives water a taste, and does not kill all microbes. But for most purposes the water will be rendered safe enough. Safest of the chemical options is iodine, and chlorine is the next most efficient means. Silver products are the least purifying—although these have the longest shelf life so are good for the occasional traveler. For travel to regions where environmental hygiene standards are very poor, I use iodine if boiling is impossible.

Alcohol is a poison. Even in its purest, Highland malt form, it is toxic, but when its origin is some still in a shack, it is likely to contain unpredictable levels of additional poisons. Be ready to face the consequences if you drink too much. Beware of spirits; distilled drinks can contain extremely dangerous toxic methanol that can cause permanent blindness. Undistilled drinks of lower alcoholic content (less than 40 percent) are unsafe if (as they usually are) they are prepared with dirty water (e.g. Tibetan *chang*). An exception is Nepali *toongba*,where boiling water is poured over fermented millet, but make sure that the water is boiling and the pot preheated. In Pakistan, one brewery is rumored to put

One hot day in Jaipur, India, I decided to try a long lemon-yellow sherbet drink that a man was selling from a rickety stall on bicycle wheels. It was ice cold and delicious, but I soon realized this was no ordinary lemonade. The bhang [cannabis] made me drunk fast and then I was hit by dramatic diarrhea that had me loitering close to the loo for the next twelve hours. Next day I was exhausted but the diarrhea had abated. In the future I would be wary of cocktails and messed-about-with drinks.

◆

Simon Howarth, 45, civil engineer, Cambridge, UK

glycerol in as a preservative for beer that is sent far from the hill station near Rawalpindi where it is produced. Anyone consuming more than one bottle suffers mild diarrhea.

Tips

➤ The newer you are to tropical travel the more careful you should be about what you eat and drink.

➤ It is not necessary to boil water for twenty minutes as recommended in many guides; this merely wastes fuel. Water that has been brought to the boil is safe enough, and boiling remains the best method of making contaminated water safe.

➤ Failing this, add an iodine-based water purification tablet or drops to the bottled water and leave for the recommended period before drinking.

➤ Adding vitamin C reduces the unpleasant taste from iodine, but this must not be added until the purifying thirty minutes has been completed.

"I eat and drink everything," said a green young volunteer on his first assignment to Bangladesh. Six months later an even greener young man was medically evacuated to Bangkok suffering from dehydration and blood loss. Hanging latrines, although illegal, are still found in rural and urban areas of Bangladesh. These makeshift bamboo pole and woven wall constructions allow the user to squat over water or rice fields and defecate, thus contaminating water and allowing dogs and chickens easy access to fecal meals. Children playing with puppies, and chickens eating scraps, share diseases from these hanging health horrors.

◆

Derrick Ikin, 53, Swiss development consultant, Maputo, Mozambique

➤ Bottled water is almost certainly safer than a suspect local supply, which has not been treated, but it is not a guarantee of trouble-free travels. Sterilizing your own water is a more ecologically sound approach.

➤ In the West, bottled water is untreated spring water from a safe source, whereas in the low-income destinations it is often treated tap water and so should not strictly be called "mineral water."

➤ International hotels will provide you with safe drinking water if you ask.

➤ In France should you want tap water, ask for a *carafe* or *pichet de l'eau*. Water quality in the European Union is usually safe enough.

➤ When staying in a more down-market place ask for a glass of boiling water. If it is hot, you know it is safe enough. In Indonesia, eating houses offer *air putih*. This is boiled water that is often served still warm; it is safe but beware of added ice which may be contaminated.

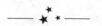

My new Brazilian boyfriend and I, on an Amazon boat journey, arrived in Alter do Chão, a place of extraordinary beauty. We saw a little of it before a violent bout of diarrhea kicked in. I spent the next few hours being propped up on the toilet by him, both of us close to passing out! Naturally, I later married that man who was so willing and able!

◆

Susanne Padilha, 38,
Brazilophile, Hong Kong

➤ If you are offered a drink—or food—which you think may be contaminated, take as little as possible; the less you consume, the less you risk stomach trouble.

➤ Concerns have been raised about the safety of using iodine to purify drinking water. Excessive use can cause enlargement of the thyroid gland in the neck, so long-term users should not add iodine to all their drinks. It is usually possible to take a range of drinks from various safe sources and a great deal should be in the form of boiled water.

➤ In 2009, the European Union prohibited the sale of iodine for use in drinking water. This was not due to safety concerns but simply because the profits on selling this cheap product would not cover the expense of the testing required for a product licence.

➤ Russian *samogon* is often made from sugar but also beet, corn, and even plywood. It is legal only for personal use; selling it is prohibited. *Samogon* may have a strong repulsive odor but, for lack of any other spirit, it is still locally very popular. The plywood version probably contains toxins.

Travelers in low-income countries can be lulled into a false sense of security by assuming that bottled water is safe water. Tests and visits to bottling plants in Nepal showed that while the majority of samples were free of fecal contamination, some rogue companies were merely bottling inadequately treated tap water. Quality control is a major issue—even leading companies lack on-site lab facilities to test for many impurities. A number rely on one-off tests in Europe at the start of production to accredit their brands. Nepal, like many countries with limited resources, has very few regulations in place to protect the quality of bottled water. This problem is not restricted to the resource-poor regions. In the USA, the Natural Resources Defense Council (1999) tested 1,000 samples of 103 U.S. brands and found that at least one-third had levels of bacteria and chemicals that exceeded the standards regulating the bottled water industry.

◆

Greg Whiteside, 41, water engineer, WaterAid, Nepal

Chapter 3

EATING RIGHT
THE PLEASURES AND PERILS OF SEAFOOD

Eat Fish—Live Longer Eat Oysters—
Love Longer Eat Clams—Last Longer

—*Bumper sticker, Delaware*

———

*T*here is good evidence that eating at least one portion of oily fish each week helps prevent thrombosis, athero-sclerosis, and consequent heart disease; fish and shell-fish form part of a healthy diet when you are staying at home, but on your travels, you need to be cautious about foods that have been harvested from the sea, rivers, or even rice fields; they can be risky. In less-developed Asian countries people use "hanging latrines" that allow feces to fall into rice fields or fish ponds, so recycling parasites and filth-to-mouth microbes. Many edible water creatures feed by filtration and so accumulate and concentrate harmful microbes. And seawater does not kill microbes so that in Peru, for example, delicious ceviche (marinated raw sea fish) was identified as a source of cholera during the epidemic of the early 1990s.

In the 1960s the people of the Philippine island of Luzon started to develop a mysterious wasting disease that caused prolonged and debilitating diarrhea. The epidemic was finally blamed on *Capillaria* worms that live in shrimps, fish, and birds, as well as in people. Locals loved eating "jumping salad" (made from shrimps so fresh they were still moving) and other raw delicacies: snails, crabs, squid, and the vital organs of fish, goats, and cows. The disease—once diagnosed—was treatable, but could have been avoided in the first place by cooking the food. Improved disposal of excreta reduced the number of people suffering from these parasites.

Undercooked seafood is risky all over the world. Even pickled raw fish from California or the Netherlands can be a source of herring worms, although these cause—at most—a transient touch of nausea and a few stomach cramps. And cases of paralytic shellfish poisoning are even recorded occasionally from the chilly waters around Britain. Symptoms begin (typically within three hours of eating shellfish) with tingling around the mouth and throat, dizziness, and a floating sensation. There can also be headache, nausea, and vomiting. The tingling and numbness progresses, and the muscles become affected so that breathing may stop altogether. In Britain, mussels eaten during the summer are usually the culprits.

From time to time tropical seas undergo dramatic blooms of tiny dinoflagellate animals that make the water look red: so-called red tides. This is signaled by the deaths of large numbers of fish and sea birds and is most common along polluted coasts. Local fishermen usually know not to catch fish during these red tides since they are poisonous. Filter-feeding shellfish concentrate red tide poisons and so must also be avoided at these times. If you must eat fish,

When the mood is right there's nothing better than a meal of sushi: raw fish with rice and other garnishes. Any good restaurant worth its reputation will serve only the highest quality ingredients prepared to eliminate all worms and parasites. If you're worried about safety, be sure to go only to restaurants that do a brisk business. That way you'll be certain all the fish is fresh.

◆

Larry Habegger, 53, writer and editor, San Francisco, California

choose individuals with clear eyes, a firm intact body that smells all right. Symptoms develop within half an hour of eating contaminated fish and may progress to fatal paralysis in twelve hours.

Ciguatera fish poisoning is more difficult to recognize; it happens when there is no obvious change in the sea. It causes several deaths a year worldwide. Like red tide poisoning, it is also due to fish accumulating dinoflagellate toxins from their food. The liver, viscera, and sexual organs or roe of large and also scaleless warm-water shore or reef fish are most likely to contain the toxin. Moray eels should not be eaten because of the high risk of ciguatera poisoning. An early sign that a fish is affected is that you notice tingling or numbness of the mouth; this progresses to vomiting, diarrhea, and cramps. Some people are left with a weird, long-term change in temperature sensation or temperature inversion when cold objects feel burning hot and painful to touch, and hot objects feel cold. These symptoms settle with time.

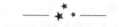

We had a great toilet in Belize, when I did a diving expedition, on a remote coral island. The bamboo hut faced the sunset, the seat opened directly into the lagoon, and the fish were very hungry. We had a few Americans visit us who were totally disgusted. But it was a conservation trip and we were very eco-friendly.

◆

Dr. Caroline Evans, 44, travel health adviser, expedition doctor, London, UK

Scombrotoxic poisoning occurs when the red flesh of tuna, mackerel and their relatives (including albacore, skipjack, and bonito), and the flesh of tinned fish such as sardines and anchovies, or others including mahi-mahi, blue fish, amberjack, and herring are decomposed by bacteria to produce histamine poisons. These toxins often cause a tingling or smarting sensation in the mouth, or a peppery or bitter taste in the fish. If you not stop eating at this point, you will go on to experience flushing, sweating, itching, abdominal pain, vomiting, and dizziness which usually goes away within twenty-four hours. This kind of poisoning is avoided by eating fresh fish or by removing the guts and freezing fish as soon as possible after being caught. The problem is most common in hot climates, because decomposition begins so quickly. Medical treatment is not necessary.

Tips

➤ Lightly cooked shellfish and sea fish can be sources of exotic parasites.

➤ If fish or shellfish may have been taken from contaminated waters, ensure that it is well cooked. For seafood from a contaminated environment to be really safe it should be boiled for ten minutes or steamed for thirty.

➤ It is dangerous to eat fish or shellfish caught during red tides; be wary of eating fish from polluted seas. When buying fresh fish, check to see that it looks and smells fresh.

The mutton fish, or pawa, although resembling India rubber in toughness and color, is a very excellent and substantial food for explorers, both European and native...[but] the sea anemone...is the most extraordinary food that ever afforded nutriment to the human body, and...in eating it, the eyes should be kept closely shut.

◆

Charles Heaphy, VC, 1820– 1881, English-born New Zealander, painter, surveyor and explorer

➤ Even in temperate climates be wary of mollusks. Eating mussels that stay closed after cooking will likely make you ill.

➤ Avoid eating very large reef fish; these may come with special ciguatera poisons.

➤ Puffer fish or *fugu*, beloved of the Japanese, is said to be outstandingly delicious but if improperly prepared is lethal. There are other fish that may also be toxic in Southeast Asia and the Indo-Pacific, so get a local cook to prepare fish for you.

➤ Strangely shaped or very colorful fish are more likely to harbor ciguatera toxin than dull fish-shaped fish.

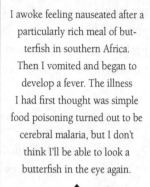

I awoke feeling nauseated after a particularly rich meal of butterfish in southern Africa. Then I vomited and began to develop a fever. The illness I had first thought was simple food poisoning turned out to be cerebral malaria, but I don't think I'll be able to look a butterfish in the eye again.

◆

Barbara Ikin, 47, development worker, Mozambique

➤ During the mating season, horseshoe crabs become poisonous; don't eat them.

➤ The sexual and other internal organs of a wide variety of sea creatures can be poisonous; it is best to eat only the flesh. And eat your sea cucumbers and fish peeled or skinned.

The delight of trips to Brittany (Bretagne) in France is the seafood. I love to buy fresh mussels or scallops and live langoustine (scampi) and cook them myself at the campsite. Seafood here is always very fresh and exceptionally tasty. The French give food a high priority so the turnover in shops and food stalls is fast, and fish and shellfish are so much fresher than you'll find in England. I think that the best seafood comes from temperate waters. The much-praised barramunda lungfish of Australia and prawns raised in the tropics cannot be compared to the seafood of Brittany.

◆

Arnold Thomas, 67, chef, Ewell, Surrey, UK

Chapter 4

WEIRD FOODS
THE RISKS OF FEARLESS DINING

Dr Buckland [popular and respected visitor to the London Zoo]
used to say that he had eaten his way straight through the whole
animal creation, and that the worst thing was the mole–
that was utterly horrible…there is one thing even worse
than a mole, and that was a blue-bottle fly.

–Augustus J C Hare, The Story of My Life, 1882

I was walking through rice fields in rural Thailand with a local engineer when a slender green snake shot across the path just ahead of us. Interested in my friend's lack of reaction to the animal, I asked, "Was that a venomous snake?"

"No, it isn't venomous and it is not good to eat either." In his eyes, this species was a complete write-off. Later I sat down to a delicious and diverse meal of all kinds of tasty tidbits of assorted textures and flavors. I asked about the slightly gelatinous black cubes in the stir-fry. "This is congealed ducks' blood,"

If you travel widely, you are going to encounter food that is unusual, strange, maybe even immoral or just plain weird. Long ago I adopted a rule for strange encounters, and it has become my motto: wherever I go, whatever people I visit, I bow to their kings, respect their gods, and eat their viands no matter what. There is nothing I will not eat or drink at least once. I am a culinary pagan, and I worship at every altar.

◆

Richard Sterling, How to Eat Around the World

my host explained, delighted I was enjoying the food. At this point I stopped enjoying the food. Thailand is renowned for its delicious cuisine and for its amazing range of foods. Shopping in Thailand is fascinating; I find myself wondering how the weird ingredients can be prepared for the table. Who, for example, might want to nibble giant water scorpions (known also as toe-biters) that seem to be a local delicacy?

Unfortunately the foods that Thais, and many of the people of Southeast and East Asia, enjoy cause some special health problems. This is because many "delicacies" are eaten raw or undercooked, and it is this lack of cooking (rather than the weird ingredients) that causes trouble. The region is well known for its great variety of parasites. There is a good range of mosquito-borne infections (two kinds of elephantiasis, dengue, malaria, etc.), and there are gnathostome worms available to those who eat freshwater crabs, raw tadpoles, frogs, and

In the Bangkok emergency room I explained my symptoms to the Thai doctor. Peering into my eye, he felt for the hard lump above my right eyebrow that had become my recent traveling companion. "You have gnathostomiasis," he announced. "It's a worm that grows under the skin, and yours is quite big so you must have had it for some time. We'll do a blood test, but there's only a 50 percent chance that it will show positive, as it only comes up at certain times, for feeding."

"Feeding!? Feeding on what?"

"Well, it lives in your soft tissues and feeds on nutrients in your blood. The usual remedy is to surgically remove it, but if you decide not to, the life span of these worms is about ten years."

He went on to explain that one gets this worm from eating undercooked shellfish here in Thailand. I had expected a sinus infection, maybe a brain tumor. But a worm living in my head? Why did I come here?

◆

Alison Wright, "Don't Eat the Shellfish," Food: A Taste of the Road

snakes. Gnathostomiasis causes lumps under the skin. Raw freshwater fish harbor *Clonorchis* liver flukes, which can cause a rather unpleasant long-lasting illness, while raw Chinese beetles and grubs may give you worm-filled lumps in the bowel, whereas raw freshwater shrimps in many regions may give you angiostrongyliasis: a nasty little worm that occasionally sets up home in the brain or eyes. Yet interestingly Indonesians are wary of some foods, especially during pregnancy: they say that pineapples cause miscarriage, squid cause obstructed difficult labor, and prawns will cause the baby to be born bottom first.

East African locusts—preferably fried in butter—are delicious, and perfectly safe to eat. On the other hand, undercooked giant African land snails carry the risk of angiostrongyliasis. Eating raw freshwater crabs in Nigeria and Zaire may give you worm cysts and abscesses in the neck. Avoid all these nasty parasites by eating your shrimps, beetles, and snails well-cooked.

The only birds known to be poisonous are three species of pitohuis, thrushlike perching birds from Papua New Guinea. They produce a powerful toxin very similar to that of South American poison arrow frogs, so that licking the feathers makes your mouth go numb and tingly. Presumably eating their flesh would do you no good, and it is unlikely that cooking will inactivate the toxin.

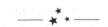

Wondering what to try for supper one day in Thailand, I was intrigued by "waterfall beef" on the menu. This was meat so fresh, and raw, that the blood was dripping off in a "waterfall." It was delicious, and fortunately this cow hadn't previously dined on tapeworm.

♦

Simon Howarth, 45 gastronome, Cambridge, UK

The people of Sulawesi, Indonesia, have some odd eating habits. The Bugis, who were traditionally pirates said to be the original bogeymen, favor offal of all sorts and especially soup made from the intestinal contents of buffalo. While this is well-cooked and thus safe, I could never bring myself to try it. Dog meat is eaten in many parts of the world, but in North Sulawesi, it is actually the local delicacy—stringy street mutt fried up with lots of chilies. As long as this is thoroughly and freshly cooked (i.e., hot), this dish should not carry any special health risks, although since these dogs are city scavengers, they are likely to be riddled with parasites; dogs are certainly known to carry *Giardia*. Fruit bats (also known as flying foxes) live a healthier lifestyle, are tasty, and pretty safe to eat. Most of us will consider dog meat an unenticing dish, but Antarctic explorers have been forced to eat their dogs, and at least one unfortunate succumbed to vitamin A intoxication—from eating dog liver. Polar bear liver, too, is dangerous for the same reason. Fruit bats (also known as flying foxes) should be pretty safe to eat although they were implicated in an outbreak of nipa virus in southern India in 2018.

Chinese engineering contractors, working near Beergunj in the lowlands of Nepal, were out hunting snakes after dark, scrambling around with torches, trying to dig them out of their holes to eat. Locals became alarmed, and mistaking the Chinese workers for dacoits (bandits), mounted an attack. The Chinese spoke no Nepali so could not explain why they were acting so suspiciously, got beaten up, and subsequently complained to the police. One way to solve the problem of rabies in Nepal is to get more Chinese contractors working in the country; they will eat all the dogs, and we will have no more rabies. Chinese eat anything!

◆

Dinesh Shrestha, 39, civil engineer, Kathmandu, Nepal

Undercooked beef, buffalo, and yak are popular dishes in many agricultural communities, but if the animals have grazed where people have defecated, the meat is likely to be contaminated with beef tapeworm. One winter in Ladakh, India, I was offered slices of yak meat as a snack. This was completely raw and crunchy from the ice within the meat; the maximum daytime temperature was around 14°F/-10°C. Even at subzero temperatures there is a risk of parasites: tape-, round-, and *Trichinella* worms survive in very severe weather conditions. Peoples of the high Himalaya love meat in most forms (there are few vegetables available), and one is often offered strips of dried (and sometimes smoked) beef or yak to chew with your drinks. I don't think these are altogether safe either. In warmer climates, armadillo tacos in Mexico and the Southwest U.S. have been blamed in some cases of leprosy in travelers. These animals undoubtedly are prone to leprosy but a little cooking will destroy the bacteria. Eat your armadillos well done, too, or choose beans.

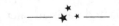

Villagers say that the water monitor is a very useful creature. You must kill the lizard and hang it up over a pot on the cooking fire so that its fat drips out. Then all you need do is apply the merest smear of this fat to the rim of the cup of your enemy or to his plate, and he will be dead by morning— and no one will know how.

♦

Lennie Domingo, 61, irrigation engineer, Sri Lanka

It can be tempting, especially when camping in a remote place, to go foraging for free foods such as fungi, berries, and salad stuffs. Take great care what you eat when traveling since some plants that are highly poisonous may resemble familiar edible plants at home; ask local advice. There is a plant, for example, which provides succulent berries to foragers in

Madagascar and looks almost identical to European deadly nightshade (*Atropa belladonna*). Consequently there are numerous hospital admissions and some deaths in Malagasy people who have consumed deadly nightshade berries in France.

Hospitable people from India and Pakistan offer paan to their honored guests. This is specially prepared from a range of ingredients kept in a beautiful box, or bought from a street vendor's stall. It is composed of a fresh green betel leaf (Piper betel), into which is put a smear

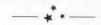

We had bat soup in Indonesia one evening, and the following day went out for a surf. My friend's stomach had already started churning, then somehow, due to some huge rise in his intra-abdominal pressure and the tight-fitting wet suit, the contents of his gut came out and managed to fire out of the back of his wet suit neck seal, into the air.

♦

Rob Conway, 27, medic, www. blueventure.org, Tooting, London UK

of lime, a fragment of areca palm nut (Areca catechu), sometimes a piece of tobacco, sometimes marijuana, and often spices. The contents are then folded and stuffed into the mouth and may be chewed or held in the cheek for an hour or so. If the mix contains tobacco, your saliva will become fiery and unswallowable which is why *paan*-chewers spit a lot, and the saliva becomes alarmingly, blood-red. Your host can modify the contents of your *paan* according to your tastes, and it is not impolite to request a less toxic concoction. There is some risk of filth-to-mouth or even waterborne infection from street-stall *paan* since the betel leaves are usually kept fresh by soaking in undesirable water and the vendor's hands are not always clean.

It is impossible to mention all possible chemical poisons that can contaminate food. However, since most naturally occurring food toxins are well recognized wherever they are consumed, local culinary habits have evolved to deal with them. Perhaps the most commonly eaten plant that is potentially toxic is the cassava; it is also called manioc. Tapioca is made from the cassava tuber. In its raw form it contains sufficient cyanide to kill, but local methods of preparation (boiling, soaking, washing in running water, and pounding) reduce the amount of cyanide to a nontoxic level. Do not prepare cassava yourself but get a local person to cook it for you. It is only a risky food during disasters or famine when there is insufficient time or fuel for traditional methods of preparation.

Eating a very sweet dish in Brazil, I asked what it was. My host said, "It's called Lady's Saliva and it's made from coconut milk, whole raw eggs, and sugar."
Then in Japan I ate dried jellyfish that had been cut into strips; it looked like elastic bands, had the consistency of elastic bands, but with less flavor.

◆

Dr. Charles Bangham, 44, medical research scientist, Imperial College School of Medicine, London, UK

In Madagascar, people eat wood-encased, cricket-ball-sized fruits of trees that are closely related to *Strychnos nux-vomica*, the source of strychnine. Although the fruits are very tasty, eating lots will bring on a headache, a symptom of mild intoxication.

Generally, though others' eating habits may seem weird they will usually be harmless. Why not, for example, add fruit conserve to tea as they do in Kyrgyzstan? The answer is that it tastes foul otherwise. And the Mozambican habit of mixing Coke with wine might seem mad at first, but when you try the wine, you'll understand.

Tips

➤ Many people who are traveling independently long term
think that they need to take
vitamin supplements. Vitamin deficiencies are most
unlikely even on the dullest
of diets unless you have very
persistent, long-running
diarrhea. Generally, those

> Shee replied, saying, thou
> mayest thanke God thou are
> leane; for they feare thou hast
> the pocks; otherwise they.
> would eate thee.
>
> ◆
>
> *John Chilton, English sailor*
> *in Mexico (1569)*

eating and absorbing sufficient calories also absorb sufficient vitamins and are unlikely to suffer deficiency syn-
dromes. Seek a varied diet, though; it is good for the sake of
both your mental and physical health.

➤ If you are in doubt about the safety of a new or weird food,
ask locals about it, and do not overindulge yourself at first.

➤ Sometimes the challenge is finding out what you are being
offered as even in translation menus can be incomprehensi-
ble. For example, we are still pondering what *husband and
wife torn lung pieces* could have been (in China).

➤ Most weird foods will be safe to eat—if unaesthetic—once
they have been well cooked and are served hot.

➤ Beef or yak raised in less-than-sanitary conditions may carry
tapeworm that will infest you unless the meat is thoroughly
cooked.

➤ Avoid eating red or brightly colored fruits and berries unless
you know them to be harmless.

➤ Never eat anything which looks like a tomato (unless you
know it is one), even if it smells pleasant.

➤ Do not eat roots, fruits, or vegetables with a bitter, stinging, or otherwise disagreeable taste. Try them with the tip of your tongue if in doubt.

➤ Consuming uncooked wild watercress in regions where freshwater is polluted carries a risk of liver fluke infestation.

➤ Seaweeds are all edible as long as you are not in a highly polluted area. The tastiest kinds are generally the pink, purple, reddish, or green types.

➤ Do not eat small wild birds in Papua New Guinea or Indonesian Irian Jaya.

➤ The liver of dogs, bears, and other carnivores is so loaded with vitamin A as to be toxic. Don't eat it.

➤ Cannibals in the Eastern Highlands of Papua New Guinea suffered slow neurological decline over months or years because they ate the brains of their victims. The

The Chinese like to be absolutely sure that their food is fresh. They like to see their chickens killed in front of them and that any seafood was alive moments before consumption. The most revolting dish I've eaten—and I am unsure how it was prepared—was a fish served up still gasping but with its flesh cooked. Drunken prawns are similarly fresh. They are put into spirit alcohol where they swim until they die, and then eaten raw. I've been given "Bull's Stamina," which turned out to be penis, "three-snake soup" (quite tasty), and boiled sheep's ear (rather chewy). One of the most dangerous foods to eat in China is the steamed meat dumplings served by street vendors. These are not kept hot enough and are highly likely to make you ill; even the Chinese are wary of them.

◆

Philip Andrews-Speed, 44, lecturer in international energy policy, Dundee University, Scotland

disease, kuru, was due to a virus akin to the agents causing Creutzfeldt-Jakob or "mad cow" disease, and appeared after ten to twenty years incubation. Such "slow virus" infections come from eating brain, bone marrow, liver, or spleen of infected animals (or people).

A farmer in the hills of East Nepal offered me a drink, but I wasn't thirsty so I declined. He was keen to press his hospitality and offered to mix yogurt with the amber fluid. I refused again and so he offered sugar, too. It was only then that I realized that the drink was fresh cow's urine. It is taken locally for its healing properties.

♦

Simon Howarth, 45, civil engineer, Cambridge, UK

While cycling across the US, we camped in Yellowstone. I took an early morning walk while a companion cooked breakfast of ham and eggs, the full works: a beautiful smell. When I returned, the camp was strangely deserted. It was like the *Mary Celest*. A grizzly had come through, knocked everything flying including the bikes, and of course grabbed our breakfast. My chums were hiding in the toilet block.

♦

Shirley Thomas, 48, transcontinental cyclist, Leicester, UK

Chapter 5

SQUAT LOOS AND
LONG-DROPS
WHICH WAY TO THE LADIES/GENTS?

Written on a wall in one roundhouse
(the military slang for lavatory) was:
"This bloody roundhouse is no good at all
The seat is too high and the hole is too small!"

Underneath was added in a different hand:
"to which I must add the obvious retort.
Your arse is too large and your legs are too short!"

—*Found by "an eccentric potter from Ireland" in a book by Alistair Mars*

*P*erhaps one of *the* most awkward experiences of traveling is to enter a place that you understood was a toilet
and then are unsure what to do or where or how to
"go." You might even wonder whether you are in the lavatory
at all. Exotic toilets come in
many designs according to local
needs, resources, and practices.
Many look like a hole in the
floor and the simplest is the
long-drop—not a giraffe doing a
poo but often slats over a simple dry pit. Such arrangements
look primitive to those of us
used to sitting on thrones to
ease ourselves, but simple squat

LOST: one Petzl headtorch in
the long-drop, Horombo hut,
Mount Kilimanjaro. Don't bother
looking down there—that's what
I was doing when it fell off.

♦

*Steve Foreman, 47, explorer,
Nottinghamshire, UK*

latrines are practical, cheap, and hygienic in warmer climates that make conventional pedestal toilets difficult to keep clean and odor-free. The best squat loos are made of porcelain, have a water seal and have a cistern to flush away your offerings, but often there is only a bucket. In parts of Asia there are hybrid toilets halfway between a squat plate design and a pedestal. There is somewhere to squat or you can fold down a seat and sit to shit.

Flush toilets might seem to be an essential part of civilized living, and indeed they have existed for a very long time. Excavations in the 5,000-year-old city of Mohenjo-daro in Pakistan have revealed flush privies and a comprehensive system of town drainage. Flush toilets are popular in the West and so development agencies often build them in remote places. A well-intentioned organization built flush toilets at the hospital in Leh, Ladakh, at 11,000 feet in the western Himalayas. During the winter the

The Tanzanian village had a toilet, a stone building with a boarded floor and a slit to squat over. Curious, I pointed a flashlight down the hole which revealed a seething mass of maggots some ten feet below. I should not have been surprised. The maggots were doing a good disposal job—there was very little smell.

◆

Yvonne Robson, 41,
veterinary surgeon, Simon's
Town, South Africa

"Are there toilets here?" I asked in my best Italian.

"Si, signore," he replied pointing to a block of public lavatories.

There was a door marked SIGNORE. "Signore means Sir, so that must be the Gents," I thought, so in I went. It was full of women! I beat a hasty retreat. Signore means Sir, but Signore also means Women! The word for Men is Signori.

◆

David White, 65, retired
headmaster, Ayrshire, Scotland

maximum daytime temperature hovers around 14°F/-10°C so the flush toilets couldn't be flushed. A dry composting lavatory would have been more appropriate, and indeed is what is traditionally used locally. These are usually a hole in the floor of a house where soil from the fields is heaped into the corner. People crap into the hole, then toss down soil on top thus keeping the toilet almost odor-free.

The excreta is naturally freeze-dried by the harsh climate and then in the spring it is dug out and used as fertilizer. My only problem with these is that they are often built into the highest point in the house, and sometimes there was a real feeling of vertigo on looking down several stories between my legs.

Locals using tropical squat loos usually use water to clean themselves, and there should be a tap or bucket for this and also to flush the toilet. Before you squat, check whether the tap functions or that there is some water in the bucket; pre-wetting the pan makes flushing easier. Some of the most disgusting loos I've used are squat toilets built for tourists in Nepal who, it seemed, were too idle to carry a little water to flush away their mess. In countries where water is scarce people are most inventive about other means of

Being tall, short-haired, with a fancy bicycle, I was obviously a man, whose insistence on using Ladies' lavatories in China was unacceptable. Women barred my way. "Go away. This is the Ladies!" they cried. "But I am a woman!" I insisted, and pushed past them. Crouching in the usual doorless cubicle, I was surrounded by gaping women. There were muffled exclamations. "Hey, get a look at this, sisters! It is a woman!" And how to tell which is the Ladies' in China? The Chinese character for "woman" looks very much like a person with her legs desperately crossed.

♦

Catherine Hopper, 37, cycling Buddhist, Manchester, UK

cleaning their bottoms. In parts of Africa, scratchy corn (maize) husks are used for anal cleaning and subsequently tossed into the long-drop. This has produced design dilemmas for development workers: latrine pits need to be bigger to accommodate all the husks.

Squat toilets are usually key-hole-shaped and some have raised places to put your feet, but it is not always obvious which way round you should face. People are baffled about which way to face in a squat toilet because there is no ideal. Generally if you are having a pee you need to face the hole and for more substantial movements you need your back to the hole. The footprint shapes in some squat toilets seem to be there to confuse the uninitiated. Before

In Eastern Europe many are marked by ∇ for men and ∆ for women; to remember which is which, put a circle for a head above each triangle, then think of women wearing skirts and broad-shouldered men.

◆

Richard Lockhart,
Šihulihi, Lithuania

In the Baltic States, they go farther and put the "heads" on the triangles for you so that foreigners will know where they stand, so to speak.

◆

Simon Cave, 61, retired transla-
tor and inveterate traveler,
Richmond, Surrey, UK

you decide what you are going to do, be warned: these toilets are designed for squatting. If you don't—or can't—squat (your knees may be seized after a Himalayan trek), whatever comes out of your tail end will splash on your shoes and lower garments. You also need to pull your pants and underwear down farther than usual. This often deposits whatever is in your pockets into the toilet. Beware: recovering these treasures will not be an attractive maneuver.

Often toilets can be identified by their stink, but it can be difficult deciding whether the lavatory you need is for men or women. In China this is often no problem since you can see the clientele inside, but in countries unused to foreigners the signs may be in another script or in code. Portuguese restrooms are variously labeled as *Sanitário*, *Mictório*, *Retretes* or just ladies or gents. *Sanitário* seems to be the term used for the automatic loos in the street while *Mictório* is a urinal and *Retretes* are bathrooms. Confusingly, *lavatório* (and also the *toilette* in France) is only somewhere to wash. And you are expected to know that H is for the gents and S for the ladies, *homens* meaning men and *senhoras*, women. In Spain the toilets are called *Los Servicios* while in Iceland *snyrting* is a toilet and *Kvenmenn* is the ladies and *Karlmenn* gents.

Some British pubs and restaurants can confuse visitors in trying to be amusing in the way they label the toilets. In Cornwall one pub indicates the door to the toilets with *YerTiz* (which translates as Here It Is). Then Neil Dixon found a seafood restaurant where they were labeled Buoys (boys) and Gulls (girls), and in Texas he was alarmed to see the Gents signed as Steers (castrated bulls) while the Ladies were insultingly called Heifers (young cows). In order to be able to identify the

Paid a visit to the loo at the airport in Ulan Bator; the signs were those silly international ones with a picture of a girl with a skirt and the man with the trousers. There I was washing my hands when an elderly man wearing the traditional del, comes into the loo, he looks around, very puzzled, looks at me wearing trousers, looks at himself wearing the long flowing skirted article, sighs, and retires into a cubicle to face his next hazard: a Western toilet.

♦

Wendy Bentall, 55, editor of the Scientific Exploration Society newsletter, Chobham, Surrey, UK

correct door in another estab-
lishment you needed to know
which breed of dog was a *pointer*
and which a *setter*. In Kerala the
code is easier to break but you
may emerge with delusions of
grandeur: toilets there are
labeled "kings" and "queens."
Maybe the thing to do is just
watch who enters which door.

Tips

➤ Before using any kind of
basic lavatory, check whether
there is water to flush it after-
wards. You may need to go
and fill the bucket yourself
before your performance.

➤ Wet the pan of a squat toilet
before use; this makes flushing easier and less messy.

➤ If there is a basket or bucket
supplied for used toilet
paper, please use it; it is the
way to keep minimalist
plumbing functional.

➤ Asians often blame toilet
blockages on use of toilet
paper, but it is usually due to
using inadequate volumes of

In South America, the pipes that
take away toilet effluent are not
designed to cope with anything
but excreta. In most pub-lic
bathrooms there is a revolting
basket full of used toilet
paper. Put yours in there,
too, rather than down the loo
or you will block the pipes.

◆

Peter Hutchison, 32,
author, London, UK

We'd been working as volunteer
doctors and were taking in a
few East African sights before
heading home penniless. We
intended to smuggle our last
few dollars across the border,
and I'd slipped our last notes
into my underpants in case we
were searched. When I retired
to the long-drop, I dropped
my pants and the dollar bills
fell into the pit. They were
gone and I was in tears.

◆

Dr. Sue Holmes, 41, general
practitioner, Cambridge, UK

water for flushing. Many travelers pour just enough water for the turd to slip down the hole, yet most lavatories need a good bucketful to make it flow smoothly as far as the sewer or septic tank.

➤ Public toilets may be scarce or squalid so make good use of facilities in cafés, hotels, bars, or restaurants when you get the chance.

➤ Always secure your pockets and your belt before entering a loo, however much of a hurry you might be in.

➤ Women will find long, full skirts are easier to "go" in than pants or dungarees; skirts cover the essentials if the lavatory door is missing or inadequate.

➤ Hole-in-the-floor toilets are designed to be used in the squatting position. Squatting down low will reduce splashing, and you will

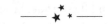

I had a dose of the runs and had to use a typically disgusting, fly-infested squat loo in a Peruvian café. As I positioned myself over the hole and dropped my drawers, there was a dull thud. My treasured Swiss army knife and its leather pouch (blessed by the Bishop of Guadalajara) had slipped from my belt. I rolled up my sleeve, plunged my arm up to the elbow into the most appalling mess and with an almighty squelch retrieved my knife. That day there was no running water.

◆

Hallam Murray, 49, who cycled 17,000 miles from California to Tierra del Fuego, London, UK

emerge pristine if you can perfect the squat! Squatting is very good for the hip joints and is the proper physiological position for moving the bowels. Practice at home you depart. Work at your balance and flexibility, and strengthen your thigh muscles.

➤ Stand clear when pulling the flush to empty the cistern. The plumbing may wet more than the pan.

➤ Some basic long-drop toilets have a cover to close the hole. Keeping this in place reduces the numbers of mosquitoes and flies inside; be sure to replace the cover after use. And then wash your hands.

➤ Tropical travelers risk two diseases from trips to the loo—mosquito bites on the bum could give you elephantiasis, and the flush-bucket and door handle could be laced with shigella. Keep well covered with repellent, don't sit for too long and wash your hands after each visit.

➤ When squatting to defecate, face the slim end of the key-hole shape.

➤ In parts of Southeast Asia, people believe they are invisible when bathing or shitting and so are not embarrassed by spectators; consequently, toilets are not always as private as you might like; ancient Romans saw going to the public latrine as a social event and would sit around chatting while moving their bowels.

Driving to Brittany, I used a hole-in-the-ground toilet with footpads; as soon as I put my feet on the pads, it flushed, soaking my new sandals. In another English-style toilet, as soon as you got near the seat it flushed and continued flushing: very off-putting when you are having a wee. Then I got soaked again entering an out-door swimming pool. I was carrying a towel and t-shirt. As soon as I put my foot in the footbath to enter, a hoop of shower jets soaked me from above. Aggh! French plumbing!

◆

Josephine Thomas, 64, retired secretary and tennis player, Surrey, UK

➤ When new to a country, ask fellow travelers how the men's toilets are distinguished from the women's; you will hear some interesting tales.

Rules for ladies using Greek "squatties":

Door (if provided) should be firmly locked.

Shorts or skirt should be removed and clutched in teeth.

Panties should be removed and tucked into bra.

Body parts should be matched to the apertures in the porcelain.

The performance may now commence.

On completion, replace clothes, flush and run like hell.

◆

Jean McRonald, 60, undertaker's daughter and sometime doctor's receptionist, Monifieth, Dundee, Scotland

---

Traveling in a truck across the Sahara Desert, we would often be sociable at evacuation time, all lined up, digging our little holes, and chatting, even while doing number twos. It reminded me of the Roman toilets in Ephesus. In places where there was very little cover, we had to squat beside the truck, and the driver—being male—thought it hilarious to drive off and leave us crouching in full view. After that we decided on a bit of female solidarity and held up sheets.

◆

Shirley Thomas, then 33, teacher taking time out, Leicester, UK

Chapter 6

WATER, WATER
DEHYDRATION, REHYDRATION

Some folks die of whisky, and some folks die of beer,
And some folks di-a-betes, and some of di-a-rrhea…

—*Anonymous*

*E*ven the wisest and most meticulously careful traveler can be struck by diarrhea, so it pays to know about its treatment. Diarrhea is an outpouring from the bowel and in its severest form can make you "go" more than a dozen times a day. It so confuses the intestine that all-essential fluids pour out of your backside or get pooled in places that are of no immediate use to your body, skulking unavailable somewhere within your abdomen. The key challenge when you begin a bout of diarrhea, then, is to replace the lost or sequestered fluid. Yet this is a time when you may not feel like drinking or eating anything. You may feel nauseated, you may even be vomiting, and your abdomen may be bloated by pooled fluid

> He looks awful: feeling dizzy, can hardly get out of bed, terrible diarrhea, splitting headache. He thinks he's dying. Could it be cholera?"
>
> ◆
>
> *Phone call from a diarrhea-sufferer's friend, Hyderabad, Pakistan*

and excess gas. So what do you do? You must drink.

During diarrhea, the stomach and intestines do not absorb fluids very efficiently: your body's normal physiological mechanisms need some assistance. Absorption is most efficient—even when you are vomiting—if fluids are taken as a mixture of water, salt, and a carbohydrate (such as sugar, glucose, or even starch). The body will be hungry for that sugar and salt, and in pulling that across the stomach wall, water will also be dragged into your bloodstream—to where it is needed. The easiest way of taking such a sugar and salt solution is to open a packet of Oral Rehydration Salts (ORS), dissolve it in clean water, and then drink a couple of large glasses after each time you open your bowels. You can drink more if you are thirsty. Many wise travelers pack a few ORS packets when they are heading for less-hygienic environments (see page 158 for the contents of my minimal medical kit). ORS packets are also widely available in little medicine shops in the low-income regions. Sometimes the language on the packet may not be one you can read but someone should be able to help—in Thailand the script is unintelligible but the solution is still called *oh-are-ess*. These packets are usually added to one glass or one liter of water (and it is important to be sure which!) but in Thailand the packet was designed for dissolution in 750 ml, which is about three good-sized glasses of water.

It must have been the food at the wedding in Bandarej, Rajasthan. My stomach started to give warning signals, I christened a rooftop, then took a rickshaw back to the hotel, stopping three times en route to empty my stomach. The doctor declared me well-and-truly dehydrated, started an intravenous drip, gave me "a little prick" in the bottom and organized a nurse who force-fed me bananas and oral rehydration solution while our local friends prayed for us. I wouldn't choose any other place to be ill in.

◆

Margaret Rivera, 59¾, recycled teenager, Lincoln, UK

Fortunately the pharmacist was helpful and anyway the only comprehensible script on the packet was "750." It is important to get the volume right; improperly made up solution can do more harm than good. If in doubt, overdilute.

If ORS packets are not available, then you can make your own sugar and salt solution. You can mix:

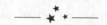

If diarrhea or heat overcome you while in India, one way to revive yourself is by taking the locally available Vijay Electrolyte (a mix of salt and dextrose) with water.

◆

James O'Reilly and Larry Habegger, Travelers' Tales India

➤ Two heaped (generous) teaspoons of glucose or sugar or honey and a three-finger pinch (less than a quarter teaspoon) of salt in a glass of boiled and cooled water.

-or-

➤ Eight level teaspoons (or four heaped teaspoons) of glucose or sugar or honey plus a level teaspoon of salt in a liter.

➤ In addition to sugar and salt you can also add a squeeze of orange, lemon, or lime juice which makes the drink taste better and also adds potassium, which is lost from the body during diarrhea and vomiting.

➤ The solution should taste no more salty than tears.

Normally you obtain a lot of fluid from your food, about three liters a day. If you are feeling too ill to eat, then you need to drink three liters *plus* whatever is disappearing down the toilet *plus* (and this is especially important if you are in a hot climate or have a fever) water losses from sweat. It is all too easy to become dehydrated and this—above all—is what makes you feel awful when your stomach is upset. Dizziness and headache can both be symptoms of dehydration, so see whether drinking makes you feel better.

Even when you are not suffering from diarrhea you must drink enough to produce three good-volume urinations a day. Allowing yourself to get dehydrated in hot climates will put you at risk of kidney stones and bladder infections.

When I have the shits, I like to take a variety of fluids, and a good light novel. I often start on a stomach-settling cola (with a pinch of salt added), but I rapidly tire of sweet drinks. My favorite is hot lemon (to which I add a little salt and some sugar), but I also like drinks made from bouillon cubes (with a little sugar added), and very weak black teas and infusions. I am always on the lookout for concoctions of clear fluids that are not sweet for these times of serious drinking.

"Simple" travelers' diarrhea can cause considerable problems if you have any ongoing medical condition or are taking any regular medication. People living with diabetes may become particularly unwell with diarrhea as the demands of the illness increase insulin requirements. And, it is all right for them to drink ORS and homemade oral rehydration solutions, despite the fact they contain glucose or sucrose.

Children and older travelers can become very unwell surprisingly quickly, because they may be less capable of maintaining electrolyte balance. Take no risks if you are traveling with kids, or you take heart medicines or you are a senior traveler. In case of severe diarrhea people who take medicines to keep their blood pressure low may need to miss a couple of doses so seek medical help early in case of problems. Make sure you are properly briefed by your physician before departure, ideally take a travel health book, too, and seek medical help early in case of illness.

Lack of understanding of the importance of drinking is the most common health "mistake." I encountered a dry-lipped American coming down from the Thorong La on Annapurna; he was so unwell and exhausted they'd put him on a horse. He looked haggard; he had diarrhea. I offered help. "You are quite dehydrated and that makes you feel bad. You need to drink liters to replace the losses from diarrhea and from breathing hard at altitude."

"I drank a quart this morning and also a glass of that oral rehydration stuff so I'm not dehydrated." But he was dehydrated. He ordered a Coke and I suggested he add a pinch of salt to it to improve absorption. "Look—I got all the salts I need from that packet...."

He misunderstood that together salt and sugar (whether in the form of ORS or salt added to cola) are a vehicle for fluid absorption, not a one-off treatment. Proper continuing rehydration would have made him feel better surprisingly quickly but he was too miserable, too unwell to listen. Yet he was feeling unnecessarily awful.

> When trekking in the Himalayas, always keep a couple of plastic bags by the side of your bed. If food poisoning sets in there is just not enough time to fight your way out of a well-done-up sleeping bag and run to the toilet.
>
> ◆
>
> *Lauren Proctor, 25, adventurer, Sedbergh, Lancashire, UK*

Tips

➤ When you have diarrhea it is important to drink lots (liters) to replace lost fluids.

➤ Any *clear* fluid (except gin) is good for rehydrating but mixtures of sweet and salt are best.

➤ Avoid milk when you have diarrhea; it can lead to a temporary allergy to milk sugar (lactose).

➤ Rehydrate with a glass of boiled and cooled water containing two heaped teaspoons of glucose or sugar or honey and a three-finger pinch (less than a quarter teaspoon) of salt and a squirt of lemon or lime juice. Brown sugar, molasses, or in India *gur* can be used instead of sugar—such "impure" forms of sugar are actually better than refined sugar since they are rich in potassium which is lost (and needs to be replaced) during diarrhea and vomiting.

➤ Add a pinch of salt to your Coke or Fanta or cordial: it sounds revolting but drinking it will make you feel a whole lot better. Lemon squash drink or hot lemon with sugar and salt added is also a good rehydration solution.

➤ Other good rehydration solutions are rice-water, clear soups, young coconut, drinks made from Marmite, Vegemite, Bovril or bouillon cubes, herbal infusions, Malagasy *ranovola*, South American chamomile tea (*manzanilla*), hot lemon and lemon tea, herbal teas, weak black tea, and very weak black coffee may also be taken. Beware of hot drinks, though: they will make you want to "go."

➤ Oral rehydration salts, ORS, are available in most countries: *Electrolade, Dioralyte, Rehidrat*, etc. in the UK, *Oralit* in Indonesia, and *Jeevan Jal* (literally water of life) in Nepal. ORS is best for children, the frail, those with long-standing medical problems, and also anyone with profuse (twelve times a day) diarrhea.

➤ When you have diarrhea, aim to drink two large glassesof clear fluid after each time you have opened your bowels and drink more if you feel thirsty. Most people will need to drink and drink.

➤ Some people find alternative treatments work well for them including homeopathy, traditional Chinese medicine, etc., but these should be taken in combination with plenty to drink. Some so-called alternative practitioners in Asia are quacks, and in Sri Lanka I have seen practitioners who called themselves Ayurvedic handing out Valium and antibiotics.

➤ Dizziness, especially on getting out of bed or getting up from a chair, is a symptom of low blood pressure. When this is caused by dehydration, the treatment is to drink *several liters* of clear fluids.

➤ Headache is a symptom with innumerable causes, but if you have diarrhea it may indicate dehydration; try drinking two liters of ORS or other clear fluids to see whether that helps.

➤ Bananas help slow diarrhea, are easily digested, and also contain lots of potassium, which is lost when vomiting or suffering diarrhea.

Before we'd started to taxi, I'd already filled six sick bags. I shouldn't have eaten the chicken salad. I only just made it to the toilet and escaped only twenty minutes later. By the time I next needed to use the lavatory, a queue had formed. Desperately I screamed "Emergency! Diarrhea!" and pushed through. Safe now, I nodded off to be awoken by a stewardess announcing, "The front toilet is temporarily out of action. Passengers should use toilets at the rear."

◆

Jo Bourne, 31,
frustrated teacher, Olney,
Buckinghamshire, UK

➤ Fluid requirements are increased to beyond three liters a day by: diarrhea, vomiting, sweating, fever, strenuous exercise, hot climate, being at high altitude, lactation, and some medications.

➤ If feeling unwell when on the bus, train, or plane, put a few plastic shopping bags (duly checked for holes) in your pocket, just in case there is no *sac vomitoire* (as they are so delicately labeled on Air Madagascar flights). Sometimes the cabin crew cannot produce them fast enough.

For the Flux—Take the chokes off a pike's head so that the teeth stick in and burn them on a tiles stone and make powder thereof and drink it with stale ale or eat it in your pottage.

◆

Unknown English author, perhaps Dame Juliana Berners, circa 1480

➤ Alcoholic drinks should never be used to rehydrate after exercise or during diarrhea. Even beer stimulates the loss of more fluid than is replaced because of excessive urination.

➤ Well or not, always avoid drinking spirits before sundown. Alcohol in hot climates leads to dehydration and sometimes even severe sunburn.

A gentleman always carries a box of matches. The sulfur in a burning match seems to be the most potent remedy for bathroom smells: strike a couple and burn them down as far as you can, and the worst of the offence will be dissipated. Do not, whatever you do, hunt in the bathroom cabinet for unused scent and spray it around; the combination of perfume and pong is an effective emetic.

◆

Serena, in The Independent *newspaper, UK*

Chapter 7

CAUGHT SHORT?
MANAGING ON LONG BUS RIDES

The boys retreated to a nearby fence. I crouched behind the largest
boulder I could find. My audience perched on top of the fence to
get as good a view as possible. When I pulled up my shorts they
were grinning at me. They hung back. I knew, with a vague sense of
humiliation, that they would examine the green mess I'd left
behind, then make full report to all their cousins and friends.

—Tim Ward, *Travelers' Tales Nepal*

———

I'd survived my first Himalayan trek and had just
returned to the civilization of Kathmandu. I hadn't eaten
much for ten days. The diarrhea had finally settled
down, but rice and lentil slop had been unenticing and my
appetite had gone. When we went out for breakfast in Thamel
though, the hot *rosti* made me drool; the portion was huge,
dripping with fat and topped with melted cheese. I hadn't
taken many mouthfuls before I realized I'd made a big mistake; this was not good food for a convalescing bowel. First
there was a brisk gastro-colic reflex, then the nausea returned,
and cramps kept me awake all night.

Rehydration—drinking liters of clear fluids—is the most
important part of treating travelers' diarrhea, or dysentery or
even cholera, but there are some other tips which will help
control your symptoms so that you do not get caught short on
the bus. The outpouring of gut contents which is diarrhea happens when the intestine is in a hurry to push out toxic mush;
often the gut is in such a hurry that it goes into spasm and

causes abdominal pains. These come and go (a constant pain is more likely due to another cause) and are often relieved by opening the bowels or passing wind. These kinds of cramps are common in diarrheal disease, but eating small quantities of bland foods can reduce them. Pure carbohydrates are best (boiled potatoes, rice, couscous, or plain crackers), and these also assist absorption of fluids if you drink plenty of water with them. Greasy or spicy foods will make cramps worse and so will very heavy meals. If you don't feel like eating, your body is probably giving you good advice: stick to clear fluids and a few dry crackers.

The physiological phenomenon called the gastro-colic reflex is something that travelers should understand. When any hot or very cold food or drink is swallowed, there is a reflex tendency for the bowels to open. Under normal circumstances this happens perhaps when breakfast stimulates your daily evacuation. When you have diarrhea, however, this reflex becomes friskier and more difficult to control so that a mouthful of ice-cold cola or a spoonful of hot rice pudding will make you want to dash to the loo. If the diarrhea is bad, the trip will have been worthwhile but because all is not well, the reflex may produce little more than a

Having succumbed first to altitude sickness and then to the dreaded diarrhea, I was resting up in a Kathmandu guest house. I was lying on my bunk one afternoon, reading, when an English trekker who had also been unwell came bounding into the room gleefully.

"How's this for self-confidence?" he said, and let fly with a terrifying English fart.

"No follow-through! No follow-through!" he chortled, leaping around the room.

♦

Rob Hosking, 35, journalist and singer of bad country songs, New Zealand

damp fart. And the big problem is—especially if you are travel-ing by bus or a light aircraft without a toilet—when this reflex strikes you may not be able to tell whether you'll have to go or whether you'll be able to hang on. If your intestines are ailing, then, avoid very hot drinks or foods or very cold or iced drinks. Aim to take any drinks at room temperature and allow food or hot drinks to cool before consumption.

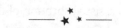

About three hours into our jour-ney from Goa to Mumbai on an overnight sleeper bus, the dodgy Indian meal hit me. I asked the driver to stop; he said, "No." As the pain got more intense I asked twice more to stop the bus; again he said, "No." I had no other choice but to shit into a carrier bag and throw it out of the window. It was no fun for me or my husband lying beside me. Have a carrier bag and toilet paper with you at all times!

♦

Jo Derrington,
Stoke on Trent, UK

On buses and coaches in the tropics you can usually persuade the driver to pull over if you need to stop, although he is not going to be very impressed if you ask him to stop every fifteen minutes. Yet even with an obliging driver, finding a place to "go" can be a problem. You can be sure that most suitable places beside the road on a busy bus route will be polluted and unpleasant and often there is little cover. I try to travel in a long loose skirt when I'm doing long bus trips in Asia or Africa so that if there is no cover at all I can just squat at the side of the road, spread my skirts, and evacuate unobserved.

Fluids and a bland diet will be all the treatment that is needed for most attacks of the shits, but if you have diarrhea that has gone on for more than three days, it would be wise to organize a stool test if you can. Medical laboratories in the tropics may have few resources but usually they are experts at stool examination. Make sure the sample is fresh—that means still warm. Almost any laboratory can manage to look at the sample under a microscope. If they see mucus or red blood cells (written RBC; a following "+" indicates RBC have been seen; "++" quite a few are present; or "+++" means that the technician has seen lots), this indicates dysentery which requires antibiotic treatment (see page 59). The kind of antibiotic depends upon the nature of the symptoms and not the laboratory result. Presence of worm eggs may be another finding, but these do not do any harm (and do not usually cause diarrhea) so you can wait for treatment until it is convenient and you trust the doctors. More sophisticated laboratories can identify bacteria and work out which antibiotic will kill that bacteria most effectively. This process takes some days, and often you will be better by the time you get the result...or you will be in the next town. A simple look under the microscope is all you need unless you are very unwell with a high fever and/or some serious problem like typhoid is suspected.

Many travelers carry antidiarrheal medicines with them such as loperamide (Imodium or Arret), Lomotil (a morphinelike drug) or codeine phosphate. These medicines do not treat the underlying cause of the diarrhea but reduce the frequency of needing to stop the bus. Personally though, I feel worse taking these drugs because those noxious microbes are kept inside for

On an eighteen-seater Nepal Airlines Twin Otter flight non-stop to Surkhet, I noticed a fellow passenger go into the cockpit to have an earnest conversation with the pilot. Soon we landed on an unfamiliar grass airstrip; the poor Japanese passenger made a dash for some bushes close to the runway, then reboarded the plane looking much happier.

◆

Simon Howarth, 45, irrigation engineer, then-resident in Rajapur Island, West Nepal

longer. Furthermore, these "blocking" drugs are dangerous if you have dysentery, if you have certain ongoing medical problems, or if they are given to a child. I don't like them unless they are taken with an antibiotic that sterilizes bugs that are partying in the gut. Generally, by taking a minimal bland diet and lots of fluids, trips to the toilet diminish, and most of the symptoms will be gone in thirty-six hours. If my diarrhea were bad, I'd delay the bus ride for twenty-four hours until the symptoms were more manageable.

Be careful about what you take from local pharmacies. Some banned drugs like the quinolone Enterovioform are still available in resource-poor countries. Medicines including chloramphenicol (sold as Chloromycetin, Catilan, or Enteromycetin) and the sulfa antibiotics (e.g.,Streptomagma) work well but they have too many serious side effects to be worth the risk in treating simple diarrhea. Do not take any of these unless there are specific indications.

The bus trip through central Ethiopia had been hard going. So had the evening meal of tough goat meat. At 2 A.M. I awoke with cramps in my stomach. The vicious dog that was tied to a high stake between me and the rough toilet shed snarled savagely. Only by making him chase in circles around the pole could I shorten his rope enough to safely edge past and eventually reach the old tin boghouse. If the dog's snarling hadn't woken the dead, then my loud explosive outpouring certainly would have.

◆

Bob Maysmor, 50, museum professional, Wellington, New Zealand

Tips

➤ The most important part of treating diarrhea is to drink large amounts of clear fluids.

➤ Drink two large glasses of ORS or other clear fluid after each bowel movement.

➤ Mixtures of sugar and salt in water are better absorbed than plain water so try adding a pinch of salt to your cola.

➤ Avoiding very hot food or drinks and very cold food or iced drinks will make a delicate bowel less troublesome so that you should be able to manage that bus, boat, or light aircraft journey without resorting to medicines.

➤ If you have diarrhea and don't feel like eating, don't eat for a day but drink lots.

➤ Bland, high-carbohydrate diets are easy to digest and are good convalescent food; these are crackers, bread, boiled rice, couscous, or potatoes.

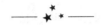

The rickety bus had jolted for hours along the mountain roads of Luzon, Philippines. When the driver drew up beside a roadside restaurant, my daughter and I joined the women, all holding toilet rolls, in a mad dash to a concrete hut. We were confronted with twelve holes in an L-shaped pattern. Absolutely no privacy, and barely room to squat without bumping elbows or bottoms!

◆

Jane Vincent-Havelka, over 60; travel writer, London, Ontario, Canada

In China, I met a fellow backpacker who'd been unable to evacuate his colon for eleven days. "Better take these then," I said, and helpfully gave him two tablets. Later I noticed I'd given him Imodium.

◆

Jeremy Garner, 28, constipated copywriter, London, UK

➤ Avoid taking medicines unless a reputable practitioner has prescribed them.

➤ Never take "blockers" like Lomotil or Imodium if passing blood with the stools and never give these paralytic drugs to children.

➤ Wait at least twelve hours before taking any "cure"—except (of course) oral rehydration.

➤ Seek medical advice if you have severe abdominal pain, can't drink, or feel very unwell.

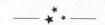

A diplomat told me this story. Chap on his way to catch a train in Delhi suffering from diarrhea soiled himself. He dashed into a shop, gesticulated to the assistant that he needed new pants, had them wrapped and rushed to catch the train. He cleaned himself up in the toilet, tossed the soiled pants out of the window, and opened the parcel to find he'd bought a shirt.

◆

Neal Robbins, 45, journalist, Cambridge, UK

➤ Abdominal pains associated with diarrhea are less worrying if evacuating or passing gas relieves the pain.

➤ Some people are left with "irritable bowel syndrome" and its associated gastrointestinal unease after a tropical trip. This diagnosis can only reliably be made after excluding Giardia infection; this is detected or excluded by laboratory examination of three separate fresh stool samples.

➤ Long-lasting mild diarrhea can be a symptom of stress, in which case the holistic, alternative therapies can be very helpful.

Hot back from a tropical trip with some unwanted hitchhikers, I visited the toilet. Diarrhea. Not confident in maintaining continence throughout the session in court, I stuffed a load of lavatory paper into my underwear, just in case. I was called to the witness box to give my evidence and noticed the court reporters stifling laughter behind their notepads. No wonder, a length of pink loo paper emerged from my trouser leg, and trailed down the steps and across the courtroom.

Steve Foreman, 47, former detective, Walesby, Nottinghamshire, UK

Chapter 8

TUMMY TROUBLES
DYSENTERY AND SERIOUS
KINDS OF INFECTIONS

The English—ah the English. They are renowned for the frailty of
their digestive systems and their preoccupation with drains and
plumbing. They have a talent for diarrhea…if an Englishman hasn't
got it, he's looking for somewhere to have it.

—Peter Mayle, A Year in Provence

—

Travelers' diarrhea is the most common gastrointestinal ailment of travelers, but you are at risk of other filth-to-mouth infections if you allow another person's feces into your mouth. Yuck, you say—never. But sometimes it is hard to avoid unhygienically prepared food, and when you do eat it, there are usually more diseases on the menu at the same restaurant. These may not cause diarrhea, but they can make you ill, and many need proper antibiotic treatment. The good news is that the prevention strategies for almost all of these fecal-oral diseases are similar. The vast majority reach you through contaminated foods, so all should be avoidable by following the advice in Chapter 1. Initially, treatments too are similar. Most bouts of diarrhea will stop within seventy-two hours, and fluid replacement (see Chapter 6) is the only treatment you will require. However, some microbes can cause quite a deal of discomfort and illness, and the following notes are to help you decide whether you need more treatment than oral rehydration. There follows, then, some details of the most common infections, or those that fascinate travelers.

Explosive diarrhea that comes on suddenly, you feel awful, often there is fever and, sometimes, visible blood in the stool, suggests bacterial or **bacillary dysentery**, usually due to *Shigella*. It definitely will ruin your day and is best treated with oral rehydration therapy and antibiotics. If you can, go to a doctor but if none is available, drink lots and consider taking a three-day course of either xifaxanta or nalidixic acid antibiotic or a dose of 1000mg of azithromycin; take medical advice before treating children. Dramatic watery diarrhea should also respond to this kind of treatment. Whether or not you take antibiotics, rehydration is still a very important part of therapy. These antibiotics will also work well for many of the microbes causing significant (that is, going more than six times a day) diarrhea in travelers, although since much of the diarrhea we acquire at home is viral, antibiotics are no help and could even make the situation worse. Don't use these treatment guidelines for symptoms you experience at home.

02.00 hours. Awoken by a twinge from my rear gunner. Chocks away! Airborne, hovering over target...fire! Payload deployed.

03.00 hours. Log alert! Sure this time my sheets would meet their Agincourt as bomb doors open prematurely. Hurling battle-fatigued cheeks onto target with thunderous roars. Mission completed...but such is the unpredictability of war (and Fijian curries), I stayed awake on sentry duty until morning. As dawn broke, lavatorial friendly fire was confirmed: my sheets were a right old Officers' Mess.

◆

Matt Collier, 26, advertising consultant, Blackheath, London, UK

Bloody diarrhea without fever is often **amebic dysentery**. This requires treatment with oral rehydration therapy and tinidazole (for five days) or, if this is not available, metronidazole

(Flagyl) tablets. Amebic dysentery tends to come on insidi-
ously, in great contrast to the
spectacular onset of bacterial
diarrheas; sufferers don't usually
feel particularly unwell.

The beautiful heart-shaped
parasite that causes **giardiasis**
swims the breaststroke in intestinal contents. As a side effect of
its activity the *Giardia* parasite
produces large quantities of sul-
furous gas which distends the
abdomen, causes cramps, and
exits as eggy belches and
foul-smelling farts. This little
beastie rarely does much harm,
but no one will want to share a
tent with you when you have
giardiasis. You may take tinidazole or, if this is not available, a
short course of metronidazole

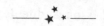

I became good at evacuating
into a yogurt pot, clenching my
buttocks, and tearing up road in
Khartoum to the clinic for a
diagnosis. A Westerner is con-
spicuous. A Westerner gingerly
carrying a yogurt pot is intrigu-
ing. A succession of foreigners
carrying yogurt pots in the same
direction is entertainment for
the locals. The doctor could give
you a rapid answer if you could
keep your insides from coming
outside. Getting home via the
pharmacy was a race against
time. Was it just a coincidence
that it also sold yogurt?

◆

*Sally Haiselden, 37, teacher,
Cambridge, UK*

(Flagyl) to get rid of it. Giardiasis can be a curable cause of irritable bowel syndrome.

Cyclospora causes diarrhea that is seldom severe, but
untreated, comes and goes over as much as twelve weeks. It
causes noticeable weight loss: of ten to twenty pounds. Treatment is with co-trimoxazole (Septran, Bactrim, etc.), but this
antibiotic is unsuitable for those who are allergic to sulfa drugs.
If this does not help, you should certainly head for a reputable
medical center and consult a doctor. It was originally confused
with blue-green algae but is now recognized as another parasite

that forms spores and so it is not eradicated from drinking water by iodine or other chemicals.

A related parasite, *Isospora*, is known to occur especially in the West Indies and tropical Africa; it causes similar symptoms to cyclospora and is also treatable with co-trimoxazole. Other parasites can turn up in stool samples but not all microbes identified by a laboratory are harmful. There is still a debate, for example, about whether **blastocystis** is a cause of diarrhea in travelers or rather only a marker of fecal contamination. Treatment with metronidazole will eradicate both blastocystis and giardia so sometimes it is worth a try.

En famille in Bali, my seventeen-year-old son got the trots and (despite all the traveling we'd done) claimed he'd never felt so ill before. I ignored his complaints and he got better— slowly. Six weeks later he was ill again, and again a month or so after that. It turned out to be his appendix. Montezuma's revenge can be more than simple diarrhea.

◆

Ro Dawson, 51, publisher, Footprint Handbooks, Bath, England

Typhoid is a nasty infection that wise travelers should know a little about. It is not particularly common, with travelers from the United States acquiring the infection at the estimated rate of only about 6 cases per million journeys. Trips to tropical Latin America and the Indian subcontinent carry the highest risk: about 174 cases per million journeys arise from returnees from Peru for example, and these figures do not count the similar paratyphoid A, B, and C infections. The symptoms of typhoid may begin with a few loose stools and then after seven to fourteen days the fever begins; there then may be constipation. Often the fever increases steadily; there is usually a headache and feeling of being unwell. After a further week, the fever has become high, making the sufferer very unwell, and by the third week there is a danger of intestinal perforation. It is a disease requiring competent medical attention and proper antibiotic treatment. Paratyphoid is a similar but usually milder illness where diarrhea is a commoner symptom. Long-lasting gastrointestinal symptoms, especially with increasing fevers, should send you scampering for a doctor. Immunization with typhoid capsules (but not the injection) provides some cover against paratyphoid. **Typhus** also causes fever, but it is acquired from tick or louse or minuscule mite bites, not the filth-to-mouth route.

Hepatitis means inflammation of the liver from any cause; symptoms are nausea, appetite loss, and intestinal disquiet, and often yellowing of the whites of the eyes and skin. Two forms get you through unsafe food: hepatitis A and E viruses, aka infective hepatitis. About a month after eating a contaminated meal, the first symptom is likely

Rumblings within made me ask my Sumatran hosts about the toilet, and they directed me outside. There I found a stinking pond with a narrow plank stretched across. Precariously fitted halfway along was a rickety old bamboo frame surrounded with cloth. I shuffled along the plank, ducked inside, dropped my shorts, grasped the flimsy bamboo, leaned back, and prayed.

◆

Vincent Ward, 39, a true believer, Chiba-ken, Japan

to be loss of appetite. There will be mild fever, aches, and pains, and then about a week later, as this all starts to settle, the yellowing becomes noticeable, the urine becomes dark in color and the feces pale. The jaundice should settle over several weeks. Complications or severe illness is rare, although it is common for sufferers to feel fatigued for many weeks after the illness has subsided. There is a chance of severe illness in pregnant women, so pregnancy is not the time to visit regions of high filth-to-mouth disease transmission. This is a viral infection—antibiotics are of no help although Ayurvedic cures in India and Nepal, and Amchi medicines in Ladakh and Tibet, seem to improve symptoms.

Polio or **poliomyelitis** is a gastrointestinal infection that can leave sufferers with a paralyzed limb. Fortunately, though, this disease is on the decline and there are effective vaccines.

Cysticercosis is the term for infestation with pork tapeworm cysts. If someone is unfortunate enough to eat pork tapeworm eggs through eating food contaminated with the feces of someone harboring a pork tapeworm, worm cysts can be laid down in the victim's muscles, under the skin, and even in the eye and brain. I have heard of this being a problem in people eating salads irrigated with raw sewage in South America: this is another reason for sticking to the "peel it, boil it, cook it, or forget it" mantra.

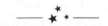

Beware of what you eat and drink just before a multi-pitch climb. When hanging 300 feet up a cliff, it is incredibly hard to get your harness off while fluid is coming out of both ends. It is even harsher if it is your mate doing this directly above you. We worked out that if you can rip a hole in the bottom of your shorts, this proves a lot easier and safer, although potentially messier, than trying to slide your harness and shorts down to do the business.

♦

Rob Conway, 27, medic, www.blueventures.org, Tooting, London UK

Cholera is a disease that scares travelers, but well-nourished, healthy adults rarely get into trouble even if they do swallow some of these bacteria. It seems to cause disease only in the debilitated or if it infects people along with other microbes. Nevertheless an oral vaccine (a drink) called Dukoral is now available in Canada and Europe and there is a similar drinkable product, Vaxchora, licensed in the US which will protect those venturing into really filthy environments since it also may give some slight pro-tection to travelers' diarrhea as well as cholera (see page 69).

There are other causes of diarrhea in travelers. Most noto-rious, perhaps, is **tropical sprue** which—untreated—can cause a persistent diarrhea that goes on for months and months. Don't let it. Seek medical help before you get run down and debili-tated. It often gets better mirac-ulously on getting home.

Finally, keep in mind that not all diarrhea in travelers is travelers' diarrhea: there are tropical causes like malaria and there are nontropical, noncom-municable causes that just happen to start while you are traveling. Sometimes it takes an expert to sort out a diagnosis so if you have continuing symp-toms, seek a medical opinion.

It's the closest I've come to being an airline pilot. Alongside the seat, in many Japanese toire, are arm rests packed with lights and buttons. Even after four years I would approach with trepida-tion. In trying to remember what the flush button looked like and testing others that looked similar, you could end up raising the seat temperature, revolving the material seat cover, or having your bottom dried with hot air or showered with jets. At one time or another we foreigners all emerged from the toilet wet down the front from "button roulette." In Japan a for-eigner is never inconspicuous.

♦

Sally Haiselden, 37, interconti-nental cyclist and teacher, Cambridge, UK

Don't take more than one course of prescription medicines without seeking a doctor's advice, and preferably at least one stool test.

Tips

➤ Most so-called "simple" travelers' diarrhea will settle within thirty-six hours.

➤ You will feel much better by keeping well hydrated: drink lots of ORS or other clear fluids.

➤ If symptoms are severe or continue beyond seventy-two hours, seek medical advice if possible. Otherwise, if no doctor is available, consider antibiotic treatment; antibiotics (with fluid replacement) are effective in treating the root cause of most travelers' diarrhea acquired in resource-poor countries and these are generally safer medicines to take than "blockers" such as Imodium or Lomotil. They also avoid the uncomfortable side effect of rebound constipation after the diarrhea subsides.

I'd eaten at a roadside meal house along with our drivers because I felt it churlish to refuse food offered to me; forty-eight hours later, my diarrhea started and I had an enforced two-day halt in a resthouse in Tirkhe Dugaa, Nepal. The "toilet" was a three-sided shelter overlooking a lovely steep-sided wooded valley. My increasing thirst and weakness made me faint while squatting and I rolled out through where the door should have been and tumbled seventy-five feet down the hillside. Kind locals carried me up to the main street. I was beyond caring as my friend cleaned me up. Then two days by wicker basket got me to a hospital and eventually continence once more.

◆

Kate Moses, 49, retired GP,
Town Yetholm, Kelso, Scotland

➤ Fever, severe diarrhea of sudden onset with frequent explosive bowel movements (twelve times a day or more), blood in the stool, and feeling very unwell are all symptoms implying you have something that is more than "simple" travelers' diarrhea. They suggest that you have a form of diarrhea or dysentery that might persist and probably needs treatment with antibiotics.

➤ I have heard it said that you can catch typhoid from filthy bank notes; that will depend upon the purposes to which they have been put and also whether they go near your mouth. Travelers, don't forget to wash your hands with soap and plenty of water before eating.

➤ It is dangerous to treat dysentery (bloody diarrhea or severe diarrhea with fever) with "blocking" paralytic medicines such as Imodium or Lomotil. They can cause intestinal perforation.

➤ Not all diarrhea in travelers is travelers' diarrhea.

➤ If you have recently returned home from a low-income region, be aware that you could still be carrying microbes that will harm

Heaven help anyone with "the runs" in Krakow Railway Station. The attendant will not allow you in until you have counted out your 3000 zloty in five or ten zloty notes. For that sum (20 cents) you get just two sheets of paper so it might be best to use the bank notes to wipe your bottom.

◆

Angela Rowe, 49, Musician/IT worker, Ystradgynlais, Swansea, Wales

1976. Arrive in Baler, on remote NE Philippines coast, after grueling drive over the mountains and am astonished to find every hotel and restaurant full, and U.S. helicopter gunships roaring overhead. They are shooting *Apocalypse Now*. Forced to eat in a dubious dive where food has been exposed, gently warming, for hours. Get my apocalypse now—explosive dysentery— but live to enjoy the film.

◆

Rowena Quantrill, 57, writer and film-goer, Bradford- on-Avon, England

others if you allow them to reach another's mouth. This is especially likely if your bowels are still a little unsettled. In these circumstances, dispose of your excreta in a toilet or bury it even more meticulously when outdoors, and carefully wash your hands before preparing food for others.

➤ Abdominal pain is common when traveling, and mostly it is mild and transient. Pain relieved by BMs or passing wind is usually benign. Appendicitis tends to start as central abdominal pain that progresses and settles in the right lower corner of the abdomen. Pains in the left lower corner of the abdomen are common in constipation and also when there is profuse diarrhea—this latter pain comes from a tired, cramped or over-stretched colon.

Many years ago I took a bus trip through Greece with some college classmates. Toward the end of the journey, I felt that I might be having an attack of appendicitis. I had severe abdominal pain, so severe I confided in a wise, old priest who was acting as a guide. He suggested a suppository.

"What for?" I asked. "I'm not constipated." But as the words tumbled out of my mouth a ray of hope presented itself. What if I was only constipated, and not dying of an unknown illness?

As soon as we got to Athens, I hastened to the pharmacy. Returning to my room, I gazed with loathing at the enormous object that I was supposed to insert into my backside. Reluctantly, yet with haste, as the abdominal pains surged, I bent to my task. Soon I was squatting over a hole in the marble floor of the bathroom, giving birth to an enormous pile of excrement that, like a mad termite colony or a volcano, could hardly be contained by the space in which it grew. Gazing with wonder at this ziggurat of colonic filth, I rose a new man, knowing with renewed clarity the meaning of resurrection.

◆

Sean O'Reilly, 53, editor and writer, Front Royal, Virginia

Chapter 9

IMMUNIZATION
AGAINST DIARRHEA
AND TRAVELERS' ILLS
PRECAUTIONS NOW AND IN THE FUTURE

My bowels shall sound like an harp.

—*Isaiah, 16:11*

————

his little book has dwelt upon those filth-to-mouth diseases that travelers risk, yet we can look forward to a time when the risks will be much less as hygiene standards continue to improve globally and because immunization will be possible against more and more of these troublesome microbes. The first time people were immunized against a fecal-oral travelers' infection was in 1896 during the Boer War when typhoid vaccine was given to protect British soldiers. It gave only partial protection in exchange for a very sore arm, fever, and often a headache, but it saved lives. That original "whole cell vaccine" was superseded only in the early 1990s by purer antigens comprising an elegantly engineered element of bacterial cell wall. These cause fewer side effects and there is also a choice of products so that now if you are one of the unfortunate 7 percent to get a sore arm after one typhoid vaccine, you can try the other.

The typhoid risk is highest in those visiting tropical Latin America or the Indian subcontinent. Travelers to other regions too might choose typhoid immunization, but this decision is dependent upon how "rough" you are traveling. It is worth noting that the injectable vaccines do not give any cover against paratyphoid fevers, but the capsules probably do. In addition immunity, although only partial, appears to last longer. The usual food hygiene precautions are still worth practicing as neither vaccine gives 100 percent protection.

An injectable cholera vaccine has been available for decades but it gave a sore arm and was rather ineffective so it was withdrawn recently. The ineffectiveness of the cholera injection and the fact that ordinary, well-nourished travelers are not at significant risk of disease from the cholera organism stimulated the World Health Organization to revise the regulations controlling international travel and cholera cover. Now international immunization certificates should no longer be demanded at border

A young woman who'd attended our travel health clinic returned from Bolivia enthusing about the value of carrying the Yellow Fever certificate that we'd given her. She was in a bus at a border crossing and some people who looked like government officials climbed aboard and began immunizing everyone; they used the same needle for all. She went frenetically rooting in her luggage, found her international vaccination certificate, and with it persuaded them that she didn't need the vaccine.

◆

Mary Kedward RGN, 49,
Director, The Travel Clinic,
Cambridge, UK

posts. Unfortunately, unscrupulous border officials have been known to extort bribes to let travelers through without certificates, even though the certificate was not required. It is often a good idea to travel with lots of official-looking health documents; sometimes they impress officials enough to allow an untroubled passage.

A cholera and ETEC vaccine called Dukoral is available in Canada, Europe and New Zealand. and has launched recently in the US too as Vaxchora. ETEC is the deviant of our normal bowel flora that is responsible for the majority of cases of travelers' diarrhea. Anyone traveling to a resource-poor country has around a 50–50 chance of getting gyppy tummy and it was hoped that this vaccine, which can be taken by mouth as a fizzy drink, would usefully protect travelers. However while it gives excellent protection against cholera, and in some studies gave up to 65 percent protection against bog-standard enterotoxigenic *E. coli* (ETEC) diarrhea it is not as efficacious as was first hoped. Interestingly, and for reasons that are not yet understood, it also seems to protect best against mixed infections of different diarrhea-causing microbes including *Shigella*, which causes spectacular and severe bacillary dysentery. Travelers to the hotspots for travelers' diarrhea and dysentery are exposed to such mixed infections and for these people this vaccine might be worth considering but other precautions are also needed for such high-risk travel. Dukoral gives two years' protection against cholera; any protection against travelers' diarrhea lasts no more than three months.

I visited a doctor in Kathmandu in the 1970s because I needed a cholera immunization before traveling from there through China. The doctor said, "I'll give you the vaccination certificate, but there's no need for the injection. The vaccine is useless."

♦

Simon Howarth, then 20, volunteer engineer in East Nepal

The situation with poliomyelitis (polio) is changing and it will be worth contacting a travel health clinic or the CDC to ask whether immunization is necessary for your destination. At the time of writing the Americas were free from the disease but cases are reported from Nigeria, Pakistan, India, Niger, Afghanistan, and Egypt. There are still sporadic outbreaks beyond these countries so it is worth checking the situation needs before any trip to destinations with poor environmental sanitation. There are still two vaccines: an injectable form which is in routine use in Europe as well as the US, and oral immunization (by bitter drops onto the tongue or on a sugar lump) is still given in some clinics. Both are highly effective.

Of all travel vaccines probably the most useful in protecting travelers from any filth-to-mouth disease is against hepatitis A virus. It has been estimated that around 5 percent of all travelers to the non-industrialized world will suffer from this kind of hepatitis and, once infected, it can leave you ill and lethargic for weeks or months. A course of two injections protects for life. It is a must for those traveling "rough". This vaccine supersedes the old gamma globulin serum which gave partial protection for a few months only. A vaccine

Travelers' health is more than just vaccinations (or shots): even if you are fully protected by all the proper immunizations, you still have to be careful of other things, especially road accidents. I have only had a few patients die over fifteen years but mostly it is from road accidents. Last year one of our patients—a most beautiful lady in her thirties—went to India to set up an orphanage. She was on a motorbike stopped by traffic policeman, and a truck ran into the bike from behind and killed her. Motorbikes are the riskiest form of transport. Tuk-tuks and rickshaws in S.E. Asia are not far behind. South Africa is another dangerous destination: one foreign tourist dies a day from road trauma, and 40 percent are pedestrians.

◆

Dr. Deborah Mills, 45,
the Travel Doctor clinics,
Brisbane, Australia.

against hepatitis E has undergone some trials but is yet to be licensed for traveler use. Various dengue fever vaccines have also been tested and one may appear in the future. Energetic research efforts are also being put into developing a malaria vaccine and one has been shown to have some protective effect in children in highly malarious parts of Africa but it is not suitable for ordinary travelers.

As immunization becomes possible against more and more infectious diseases, vaccine combinations are being launched to reduce the number of injections before any trip. When the different components have different booster intervals (as with hepatitis A and B, and also the new hepatitis A and typhoid), immunization schedules become mindbogglingly complex. Allow your travel clinic nurse plenty of time.

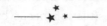

For the bloody menson—Take a herb called centynodum that is to say a hundred knots and boil this herb in water until it is soft and put your feet in it, not too deep but about to the middle of the foot for if you put your foot over the ankle bone it will constipate you so severely peradventure you shall never go to stool.

◆

Unknown English author, possibly Dame Juliana Berners, circa 1480

There are increasing concerns about the recrudescence of tuberculosis (TB) globally, and I am often asked about whether the Bacille Calmette-Guérin (BCG) intradermal immunization is useful and protective. It does offer some protection but mainly against the two serious forms of the disease (TB meningitis and miliary TB). It is less effective for the most common forms of TB. In addition, giving BCG makes the diagnosis of TB more difficult for doctors. American doctors tend not to give BCG, while British and Dutch doctors will often recommend it for extended trips to non-industrialized countries. Go with the advice of your doctor at home.

TABLE: IMMUNIZATIONS RECOMMENDED FOR MANY TRIPS TO RESOURCE-POOR COUNTRIES

Disease	Booster interval	Route of disease transmission	Notes
Tetanus	10 years	Dirty wounds	Wise for travelers and nontravelers alike
Diphtheria	10 years	Airborne	Especially for Eastern Europe and Western Asia
Polio	10 years	Filth-to-mouth	Still necessary for some trips to the low-income regions
Hepatitis A	lifelong	Filth-to-mouth	Especially for Central and South America and the Indian subcontinent
Typhoid injection	3 years	Filth-to-mouth	Especially for Central and South America and the Indian subcontinent
Typhoid capsules	5 years	Filth-to-mouth	As for typhoid injection but capsules give some protection against paratyphoid too
Cholera	2 years	Filth-to-mouth	Drinkable vaccine. Ordinary travelers are not at risk of cholera

(Continued)

Disease	Booster interval	Route of disease transmission	Notes
Yellow Fever	lifelong	Mosquito (dusk and day bites)	For much of the tropical Americas and parts of Africa
Meningococcus (bacterial meningitis and septicemia)	3 –5 years	Airborne	Especially for Africa in northern hemisphere winter months
Rabies	3 years	Animal bites	Needed for long trips to remote places
Hepatitis B	About 5 years	Dirty hypodermic needles, unsafe sex	Wise for long-term expatriates, in case of substandard emergency medical treatment
Tuberculosis (TB)	Once only	Airborne	The BCG immunization tends to be given by British and Dutch doctors but not in America or much of the rest of Europe
Influenza	Annually	Airborne	For at-risk travelers: asthmatics, diabetics, seniors
Pneumococcus	Once only	Airborne	Especially for at-risk travelers: with sickle cell disease or no spleen but may also be given to others
Japanese encephalitis	2–3 years	Mosquito (dusk and night bites)	Mainly for development workers assigned to rural Asia
European tickborne encephalitis	Annually	Ticks in Europe and central Asia	For summer bush-walkers, orienteers, and campers

Tips

➤ The filth-to-mouth diseases (diarrhea, dysentery, typhoid, hepatitis A, etc.) are most prevalent in tropical Latin America and the Indian subcontinent, including Nepal and Bhutan. It is best to be fully immunized against all possible filth-to-mouth diseases if visiting these regions.

➤ At present vaccines are available against several filth-to-mouth diseases (typhoid, hepatitis A, and polio), and they are recommended for many journeys. However, new vaccines will soon emerge and it is worth seeking up-to-date information from a travel clinic or from the CDC on what is available and needed.

➤ Allow plenty of time to organize your pre-trip immunizations—six weeks or more.

By the time my bowels start to move I realize that here in the center of Szeged there is no bog in sight. I discover a small cemetery and squat behind a large gravestone. A small dog appears. Where is its owner? I'm still squatting: don't want to put my head above the gravestone till I'm all done up. Inspiration! I rummage for the sausage I'd intended for supper. The dog wags its tail enthusiastically. I launch the sausage into the air and it lands twenty yards away. The dog rushes after it and I hurriedly squeeze out the last crap. Quick wipe with a few leaves and some grass, zip up, pull on my rucksack, and emerge to see a rotund woman in her fifties trying to disengage the sausage from her dog's mouth. Perhaps her husband will get sausage for supper.

◆

James Carnegie, 36, poet and failed environmentalist, Cambridge, UK

➤ Immunizations are worthwhile but do not protect you
   from all diseases, nor do
   they protect from the most
   common cause of death
   abroad: accidents.

➤ Finally remember that
   immunization only protects
   against a tiny minority of
   travelers' health risks. To be
   sure to survive your trip:

- Remember that emer-
     gency services and health
     facilities may not be as
     good as at home; don't
     take risks.

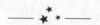

I arrived in Madagascar from
Thailand via India and Kenya,
and the health authorities in
Antananarivo wanted to keep a
close eye on my health. Maybe
they thought I'd imported cholera from India and yellow fever
from Nairobi. To make sure I
reported to the Health Ministry,
they confiscated my immunization certificates, and only reluctantly returned them the day
before I left Madagascar.

◆

*Simon Howarth, 45, irrigation
engineer, Cambridge, UK*

- Think safe; foresee and
  forestall accidents.

- Play safe on any sexual encounters.

- Be properly insured for all you plan to do.

- Protect yourself from biting insects, especially from dusk
  until dawn.

- Fair-skinned adventurers should avoid excessive exposure to the sun, especially during the middle of the day.
  Skin cancer is increasing among Caucasian travelers.

In Madras we made our way among groups of men repairing nets in the sand, watching our step to avoid the steaming piles of human excrement (the beach is "dirty," we'd been warned), exchanging smiles and conversation with fishermen. A man wiping his behind in the surf rolled his lungi back to his knees and leapt up as we passed, saying "How are you, what is your name?" Rather than shake his proffered hand we tented ours in the traditional Hindu greeting, said *"Namaste"* ("I bow to the divine in you"), and continued our stroll.

◆

—*James O'Reilly and Larry Habegger,* Travelers' Tales India

During the COVID-19 pandemic, only one person was allowed in our school toilet block at a time. To signal whether someone was in the toilets or not there were two squares on the floor outside. One had a 1 in it; the other a 0. If there was a teddy bear in the 1 square that meant the toilet was occupied or someone was using the sinks. If it was on 0 it was free. When you went inside you had to kick the teddy from 0 to 1 and when you left you kicked Pooh Bear back to 0.

◆

—*Deri Cairns-Howarth, 17, keen rugby-player, Aberystwyth, UK*

Chapter 10

COPING WITHOUT PAPER
TIME-HONORED METHODS
FOR KEEPING CLEAN

Cleanliness is half of the Faith.

—Koran

*I*n cosmopolitan meeting places, like airports and universities, one can find evidence of others' difficulties in unfamiliar lavatories: footprints on the toilet seat betray a squatter struggling with our strange Western facilities. Local experts using their own familiar squat loos usually use water to clean themselves, and so their toilets are furnished with a tap, jug, bucket, or even sometimes a bum-gun spray for this purpose. Anal cleansing with water is an excellent and hygienic habit which most Westerners find quite revolting, yet citizens of warmer countries find our habit of using paper instead of water incomprehensibly uncivilized and dirty. Just think of all that unsightly used toilet paper! The River Cam that flows through Cambridge in England was once the city's sewer and, while on a tour of Trinity College, Queen Victoria asked "What are all those pieces of paper floating down the river?" With great presence of mind her guide, Master

After living in Pakistan, I use water in the wilds. This has two advantages—you don't have to carry toilet paper and there's no messy paper left behind.

◆

Phil Brabbs, 42, teacher trainer,
Plzen, Czech Republic

of Trinity Dr. Whewell, replied "Those, ma'am, are notices that bathing is forbidden."

Yet toilet paper is a recent invention. The first, Gayety's Medicated Paper, was produced (in England) in 1857 and came in flat packs. It was a product for the rich, and one that people were embarrassed to purchase; it was kept out of sight under the counter and euphemistically called curl papers. Toilet rolls appeared in 1928, and soft paper was introduced in 1932 but it was unpopular at first. As a child in the early 1930s in London, my mother tore up squares of newspaper to be left in the lavatory for bottom-wiping; it becomes softer and more absorbent, she says, if you crumple it before use.

Whatever you think of the technique, if you are traveling for months in a remote toilet-paper-free zone, anal cleansing

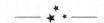

Cleaning oneself after defecation, throughout South Asia, involves…water…brought to the latrine site in a pottery, metal, or plastic vessel, called a bodna that has a spout, much like the spout of a teapot, and holds two to three liters of water. The use of this vessel is restricted to this one purpose. The…cleaning of the anal region occurs immediately after defecation. Water is poured from the bodna into a cupped left hand and then swiftly carried to the anal region. This process involves some skill and is taught to small children at an early age. After [that the left hand is] rubbed with soil…the individual pours water from the bodna onto the left hand for rinsing.

◆

Dr. Bilqis Hoque, et al., Journal of Tropical Medicine and Hygiene (1995)

with water is a skill worth mastering. Consider the trees you are saving: in a lifetime, the average Westerner's toilet paper use consumes about twenty-two trees. The technique involves using *lots* of water; pour it directly onto your bottom to flush all the unpleasant lumpy stuff and then there is little need to use your fingers. In a warm climate washing like this is considerably more hygienic than using paper and will help reduce thrush and fungal infections around the groin: the damp area dries quickly without a towel. If you are up in the mountains, wiping off excess moisture with your hands speeds the drying process or you might need to use a small towel. But one warning: anal cleansing is best done while in a deep squat. It is difficult to wash like this when on a conventional pedestal toilet. The usual result is that you will pour water all over your pants. I am now fairly comfortable with this technique although my left-handedness caused me some dilemmas at first. I wondered whether I should follow the local convention of reserving the left hand for the bum and the right for food: when traveling in Asia, it is good to be proficient at eating rice and sloppy vegetable curry without cutlery. At first I rinsed my bottom with my right hand and stuffed rice into my mouth with my left, until

In a remote village in Chin State, Myanmar (Burma), I was ushered to a toilet. My hostess must have decided that I could use some paper. Over the gap above the door she threw in a few sheets of thick white photocopy paper: not very pliable, not readily biodegradable. I folded it, shoved it in my handbag and used water.

◆

Glenys Chandler, Ph.D., 55, community development specialist, Melbourne, Australia

Best of both worlds: moisten toilet paper in water and then use it to clean yourself. Repeat if necessary. Pat dry with toilet paper only. In India and Nepal most people, after using the bathroom, do not use soap and water, but dirt from the ground to clean their hands, and then rinse their dirt-smeared hands with water. Dirty dishes too are "cleaned" with dirt or ash.

◆

Rajendra S. Khadka, editor of Travelers' Tales Nepal

one dignified old Indian lady took me to one side. "Look, my dear...I don't mind, but here in India orthodox people will be shocked if you eat using your left hand. You do know what we Indians do with our left hands, don't you?" Thereafter I washed my bottom with my sinister hand and was less than dexterous in conveying rice to my mouth with my clumsy right hand. In Pakistan I was told to be careful of holding out an outstretched hand when indicating how many items you want to buy in the market. Apparently holding up a hand palm forward, fingers outstretched in a way you might when requesting five bananas is incredibly rude. To a Pakistani it says "you are the fifth son of the fifth wife" and Muslims are only allowed four wives. Making this gesture with the left hand further increases the insult to the recipient's ancestry.

Interestingly, although scouring the hands or plates with dirt or ash seems unhygienic, research in Dhaka published by Dr. Bilquis Hoque and colleagues (reported in *Journal of Tropical Medicine & Hygiene* 98 - 1995 and in *Public Health* 109 -1995) has shown that cleaning (by scouring) the hands with mud or ash and plenty of water is bacteriologically fine: just as good as with soap. The scientists assessed the numbers of fecal

In the early days of Nepalese tourism, the guest houses of Namche Bazaar had a certain reputation—or at least their loos did. I was last there in January 1983, when for several weeks the temperature hovered around freezing. By the middle of the month, frozen brown stalagmites had started to rise through the holes in the outside loos. Tales abounded of visitors doing battle with these burgeoning beasts; but to my enormous relief I found that my landlord had thoughtfully provided a small hammer.

♦

John Pilkington, 50, explorer and author, Winchester, Hampshire, UK

bacteria remaining on hands after using different washing agents; mud, ash, and soap all achieved satisfactory levels of bacteriological cleanliness. It is a useful, cheap means for poor villagers (and ill-equipped travelers) to wash. People may prefer soap for cosmetic reasons, but the poor cannot afford such luxuries.

It is crucially important for travelers in less-hygienic regions to take special care in washing their hands before eating, and of course after defecating. It is not always possible to find soap and running water in the place of easement, which is perhaps, why door handles of squalid toilets will be hopping with virulent microbes. Whatever washing agent is used, whether it is soap or mud or ash, it is the rubbing process that gets rid of microbes and hands must be rubbed together at least ten times. Good, effective hand washing takes around 20 seconds and requires plenty of water. Alcohol hand gels are far less effective in removing bacteria and rinsing with water alone does not produce effective cleaning. Similarly, campers can scour plates clean with mud or ash, then rinse and dry them in the sun; this will make them clean enough and safe enough.

Even the well-adapted adventurer might find herself in the great outdoors without paper and without water, so then what

Traveling the back roads to Timbuktu, an occasional store may have a toilet roll lurking on the top shelf—retrieved by a rickety ladder and a storekeeper muttering "tourists" as he blows the thick layer of dust off. Failing this—and if dysentery strikes—you may have to say "When in Rome…" After three weeks of using your left hand for previously unimaginable tasks, it becomes easier, but you may need to carry extra water for your toilet ablutions.

◆

Fran King, 37, trans-African cyclist and veterinary nurse, Hornchurch, Essex, UK

do you do? The Roman soldiers used sponges soaked in vinegar, while more refined citizens used wool soaked in perfume, and rich ladies used ostrich feathers. Excavations in English medieval cesspits (we English have the strangest hobbies) suggest that people then used various materials to wipe their bottoms: the poor used leaves, moss, or stones while moneyed people cut up their worn out clothes. And even today, in poor communities, practices are similar. Where water is short, people use leaves, dirt, or stones. If you too have to resort to wiping with leaves, though, be careful what you use. Some leaves sting or irritate and others may harbor a noxious insect.

Ancient Romans revered two deities of the toilet: Crepitus was the god of the loo and Cloacina the goddess of the common sewer. Roman public lavatories, called cloaca in her honor, contained shrines where people made offerings to Cloacina. If such facilities were not immediately available, rich Romans

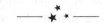

Mobile toilets on tricycles can now be found in the city of Taiyuan, Shanxi province, China, where they are popular in crowded places like the railway station or public squares. Their designer, Xue Mingyuan, a former peasant farmer, said that the toilets are convenient for pedestrians and the floating population of migrant workers, who have difficulty finding a toilet in large cities. They are one-fourteenth the cost of a traditional free-standing toilet.

◆

*Found by Tim Burford
in the Guardian*

In one town in India, the only loo available was a men's urinal and I was wearing dungarees. While struggling to "go" I looked up to find the windows crammed with peering faces. Traveling women shouldn't wear dungarees.

◆

Dr. Ildiko Schuller, 38, pediatrician and mother, London, UK

would snap their fingers, and a slave would bring a special cloak and potty for immediate relief. A similar system was available to the public in Tudor Edinburgh. Men wandered the streets crying, "Wha wants me for a bawbee?" and for that fee (a bawbee is a coin worth three Scottish pennies) you would be provided with a bucket and a tentlike cloak. That is how a problem was solved in Britain. In parts of Southeast Asia (e.g., Indonesia) people believe—or at least act as if they believe—that they are invisible while they are "performing"—they aren't embarrassed if you aren't. Whereas in Nepal, people say, "The person witnessing someone shitting is more embarrassed than the shitter."

I had lived in Nepal several years before my Nepali language skills were good enough to dare ask the low-caste attendant in the Kathmandu airport lavatory about the facilities. In the main part of the Ladies, opposite the wash basins, were ceramic plates with a tiny drain hole. The attendant, amused by my ignorance, gathered the enormous folds of her sari around herself

Your last piece of toilet paper. Fold it in quarters and tear off the corner so that you have made a small hole in the center of the square. Keep this small piece. Insert your left index finger through the hole, wipe the mess off your bottom with the same finger, then wipe the mess off your finger by wrapping the toilet paper down around it as you slide it off. Remove remaining excreta from under your nail with the retained corner. Find some water to wash!

♦

Paul Goodyer, 43, managing director of Nomad Travel Pharmacy, London, UK

and squatted over one to demonstrate that it was a urinal: saris, lungis, and sarongs nicely preserve feminine modesty even while urinating in the public part of the lavatory; the trick is facilitated by the absence of underwear. These Eastern-style facilities were only provided in the domestic terminal; apparently planners expect all international travelers to cope with Western pedestal toilets.

Tips

➤ Wise travelers carry a small supply of toilet paper, or learn to bottom-wash.

➤ Wet wipes can be useful, especially if you have a particularly messy diarrheal bowel action. They are also useful for cleaning your hands if there is no water about, but be sure to wash with soap and water when you can.

➤ Alcohol gels do not clean the hands nearly as effectively and soap and plenty of water.

➤ If traveling long term, learn how to clean up with water and no paper. If you are a novice in the technique, completely remove your lower garments so that they don't get wet. Use lots of

On the Sarimanok sailing canoe we had no lavatory but hung with our posteriors over the sea. On the rare occasions when the sea was calm, we could sit on the paired outrigger supports. Sometimes the sea came up to dunk our bare bottoms, and Steve remarked while in motion "Hey, this is like going in a washing machine. It cleans you up lovely!"

♦

Sally Crook, 47, nutritionist and author of Distant Shores: By Traditional Canoe from Asia to Madagascar

Carry a small bottle of eucalyptus oil and a light cotton scarf when traveling. Then before entering that unsanitary toilet, just dab a little of the oil onto the scarf and pull the scarf up over your mouth and nose; this helps disguise the odors that make you dry-retch.

♦

Kellie Primmer, 29, travel consultant, Victoria, Australia

water and pour it straight onto the messy area with the jug or mug provided.

➤ In desert areas you may need to carry extra water for anal cleansing.

➤ A squirty water bottle can come in useful after an unexpected shit.

➤ The average American uses three rolls of toilet paper a week and this is responsible for a great deal of trees being felled.

➤ Offering people things with your left hand will give offense in many cultures since the left hand is reserved for anal cleansing. Experts keep their left hand for the anus and their right for eating and shaking hands. Left-handed travelers may cause unintended offense by handing people things with their left hand.

——— ✦ ———

All kinds of toilet accessories are available in Japan including antiseptic wipes, seat covers, and pocket-size sprays in case you leave a nasty smell.

Toilets come in four grades:

Traditional—a basic urinal set in the floor, paper usually not provided

Basic—similar to the loos we know at home

Deluxe—this is the most common; it has a heated seat

Super Deluxe or "Full Service"— with lots of buttons and dials that I've never dared use, but one makes the sound of a flushing toilet, and so disguises any embarrassing sounds you make. The plumbing is designed so that the water you wash your hands with is used to flush away your "doings."

◆

Jo Surtees, 29,
wandering English teacher,
Iwate-ken, Japan

➤ Take care what you use to wipe your bottom; some leaves sting, others will cause irritation. Avoid wiping your bottom on any "hairy" leaves. These will definitely cause you grief.

➤ Scrunching up hard paper makes it slightly more soft and absorbent and better for wiping your bottom.

➤ Those with sensitive noses should travel with some strong-smelling potion to disguise those foul loo stinks. Carry matches.

Aid workers in Nepal and India have assisted farmers to construct biogas plants which use a mixture of animal waste and water (slurry) to generate methane gas; the gas is used to cook on or for domestic lighting. Peoples of this region have been cooking on cow dung for thousands of years, but it has taken a little more work to persuade them that adding human excreta to the slurry is also acceptable. Biogas plants are now popular since they reduce the amount of time needed to collect fuel-wood and they may help reduce cutting of the forest.

◆

Rajendra S. Khadka, editor of Travelers' Tales Nepal

Chapter 11

WOMEN'S UNMENTIONABLES
CHALLENGES AND SOLUTIONS
FOR FEMININE TRAVELERS

ANNOUNCEMENT

For the sake of the holiness
And our safety, we kindly request
Women being menstruation can
Not to enter the temple

—*Seen in Bali, Indonesia*

———

*W*omen who venture beyond the realms of flushing toilets have a few special challenges and most will agree that the biggest is coping with menstruation.

In the 1960s Dr. Hallberg and fellow medical researchers published an account of their studies of 476 Swedish women in Göteborg. They'd collected all their sanitary pads and tampons over several months, and thus calculated actual blood losses. They concluded that an "average" woman—whatever that is— loses just 35 to 40 milliliters of blood with each menstrual cycle. That approximates to only about eight teaspoonfuls spread [as it were] over four or five days, which doesn't sound like much, does it? Interestingly women can't judge whether their loss is heavier than average or lighter. Women who complain of excessive blood loss and are judged by their physicians as problem heavy bleeders often still only lose less than 100 milliliters over several days. It is puzzling then just how messy, embarrassing, and incapacitating our monthly bleeds can be.

Lots of people and many physicians have ideas about suppressing menstruation to make life for intrepid women easier, but if you do decide to take medical advice and allow physicians to play with your hormones then make sure that you organize this several months before you head off into the wilderness: any new method can cause spotting in the first two or three months. Many women conclude that it is best to simply go traveling with unmolested hormones but pack plenty of sanitary protection carefully stored in waterproof containers, for menstruation often becomes lighter with all the changes wrought by travel.

Disposable towels and tampons aren't the only solution, of course. There are washable products and also devices to collect blood such as the Mooncup (see www.mooncup.co.uk) or the DivaCup. These are small soft cups with a stalk, which fits in the vagina to collect menstrual blood. It is an environmentally preferable alternative to regular sanitary protection, and removes the need to carry disposables where they might be difficult to obtain and might pollute the local environment. You do need clean hands to take it out and empty it though, as well as somewhere to dispose of

Disposal of sanitary products and condoms may be a problem for travelers. These should not be flushed down any toilet anywhere. The UK has a "Bag It and Bin It" campaign, supported by water companies, and sanitary product and condom manufacturers. Burning sanitary products is difficult, requiring a decent fire, not just a cigarette lighter; they don't compost well so it is unkind to dump them in long-drops.

◆

*Jean Sinclair, 39,
expedition nurse and scientist,
Cambridge, UK*

the still-liquid blood and access to water to clean the Mooncup before reinserting it; this will be a challenge in many regions.

Perhaps the solution is to use both conventional supplies and such a device depending on the facilities available to you at the time. Otherwise washable pads might be useful; these are available from many online baby product stockists.

If I were planning a major mountain ascent, though, I'd arrange to stop my menstrual periods altogether with depot injections of DMPA (medroxyprogesterone acetate, also known as Depo-Provera and Megestron). This contraceptive method is back in vogue with young British women since the injections (into the buttock) are only required four times a year. Furthermore after two or three shots most women using this method stop menstruating and the vast majority of users welcome the absence of their monthly "curse". Once settled on this method too, breakthrough bleeding is unlikely if travelers' diarrhea strikes. Despite the fact that this progestogen hormone method appears to change female physiology, Depo is also safer with regard to DVT risk

In the Okavango delta, the guide showed everyone how to take a dump by leaning against a tree—otherwise you were prone to fall over in the marshy bits.

◆

Dr. Caroline Evans, 44, travel health adviser, expedition doctor, London, UK

Local women in many regions use strips of cloth to catch menstrual blood. I visited a nursing college in Nepal and, while being shown around by the Director of Nursing, we noticed a hillside covered with colorful scraps of freshly laundered cloth all laid out in the sun to dry. My hostess grumbled, "I keep telling those girls they must throw away these, not wash them. It is most unhygienic, and unsightly also!"

◆

Dr. Susanna, 25+, past Nepal project coordinator Save the Children, London, UK

when compared to the birth control (aka the combined oral contraceptive) pill (see next page). Progestogen implants such as Implanon or Nexplanon can achieve similar results (as well as giving contraceptive cover for three years). Alternatively, and for those who want control at short notice, women can take norethisterone tablets three times a day; this progestogen will suppress menstruation for as long as the tablets are being taken but it only delays rather than avoids a bleed. This is used a great deal when women realize that their monthly bleed will come during a honeymoon or other important romantic time, or when "purity" is required for religious reasons.

Not all traveling women, of course, need to worry about menstruation. Many will travel while pregnant. In many countries, foreigners who are obviously pregnant will find themselves treated like honored guests and certainly they will be mothered and well looked after. Other women demonstrate exhibitions of touching sisterhood when encountering an expectant mother. Seats are given up and the burgeoning belly patted affectionately. Everyone has ideas

A friend of mine peed in her ski suit hood when she hadn't pulled it down far enough. And we saw a German lady, naked from the waist down, crouched on her skis mid-pee as she went backwards down a slope, screaming. Always take your skis off if you pee behind a tree on the slopes.

♦

Dr. Caroline Evans, 44, travel health adviser, expedition doctor, London, UK

about what pregnant women can and can't do though. Indonesians are wary of some foods, especially during pregnancy: they say that pineapples induce miscarriage, squid causes obstructed difficult labor, and prawns will mean that the baby will be born bottom first. Pregnant women are at a very real increased risk of catching malaria when exposed to malaria mosquitoes and, once

infected, are more likely to die from the disease—and/or to lose
the fetus. Trips to sub-Saharan Africa, where malaria is a significant risk, are unwise during pregnancy and venturing into
less-than-sanitary parts of Asia and tropical Latin America carries the grave risk of severe hepatitis E infection for the pregnant
woman. Best to save trips to
these regions until after the child
is born.

All women need to be aware
that there is an increased risk of
a blood clot forming in the legs
during immobility in the sitting
position for more than five-and-
a-half hours. This can lead to
so-called travelers' thrombosis
or "economy class syndrome."
This doesn't only happen on
long-haul flights but also occurs
after bus or car trips of more
than five-and-a-half hours.
Older women are at higher risk
than women under fifty; women
taking estrogen hormones for
contraception or as hormone
replacement therapy are at
higher risk than those taking
progestogen only or nothing;
and women who are pregnant or
who have had a baby in the past

On six-week expeditions to
Himalayan and Arctic regions,
128 women aged 16 to 20 found
that taking the combined oral
contraceptive pill specifically to
prevent menstruation wasn't
worth the trouble. Those who
didn't take the pill said that their
bleeds were less frequent, less
painful, and shorter than at
home, although less predictable.
Some of those who did take the
pill were caught out without
sanitary protection by unexpected bleeding. Diarrhea, too,
can cause the pill not to be
absorbed properly, resulting in
breakthrough bleeding—an
unwelcome addition to diarrhea!

◆

Jean Sinclair, 39,
expedition nurse and scientist,
Cambridge, UK

ten days are at considerably (60x) increased risk. People with
close blood relatives who have experienced clots are more
likely to experience one themselves. Protect yourself by getting

up out of the sitting position every hour or two, wearing flight socks, and also perform calf-flexing exercises that mimic walking.

Finally women are more prone to urinary tract infections than men because the female bladder is just too close to the outside world. Tropical travel can increase the risk of such bladder infection especially if women don't drink enough. I've met many who—because they feared venturing into squalid or unfamiliar facilities—would deliberately keep themselves dehydrated and thus avoid the need to pee. This is unwise and unhealthy. Everyone needs at least three good-volume, light yellow-colored urinations in twenty-four hours. Female tropical travelers, especially those who wear tight pants, more prone to thrush and should probably pack a remedy.

Tips

➤ Women's clothes are generally poorly designed for comfort and convenience and never have enough pockets. When flying I usually travel in a shirt with breast pockets so that I can keep my passport and a pen handy.

➤ The new activities that happen when traveling can have the breasts bouncing in an unaccustomed way. Avoiding underwire bras will help

My work in Nepal often involved going on field trips to remote villages where sometimes the water source had dried up and there was never a loo. Sometimes the only privacy to allow me to change tampons was after dark, as trips to crouch down in the maize in daylight were invariably accompanied by a small band of onlookers.

◆

Dr. Susanna, 25+, past Nepal project coordinator, Save the Children, London, UK

reduce breast pain in active
women—sports bras are a
good investment. Similarly,
well-rounded thighs can rub
together uncomfortably if on
a walking vacation; explore
sports clothing that will protect from chafing. Moisturiz-
ing creams are worth
packing.

➤ Female shapeliness means
that sleeping on a hard surface can be uncomfortable;
tying a sweatshirt or some
other thick garment around
the waist will make for
sounder sleep.

➤ Urinary tract infections
(UTIs) aka cystitis are
common in traveling women
and are signaled by pain
right at the end of urination.
If far from a clinic, try taking
lots of extra drinks and add a
teaspoonful of bicarbonate of soda (aka baking soda) to
each big glass of water. In some destinations cooking ingredients are easier to find than a doctor.

➤ Women taking estrogen in their contraceptive pill or as part
of hormone replacement therapy are at increased risk of a
blood clot during or within ten days of a flight of more than
five-and-a-half hours duration.

— ⋆ ⋆ ⋆ —

I'm often surprised at the
women travelers who don't
know about panty liners. Many
of us have used them for years,
and find we only need two extra
pairs of briefs for even a long
trek as they keep clean for days.
Bring enough for one per day,
plus extras for accidents, or for
added protection during a bout
of diarrhea. They come in various lengths, and the most convenient are individually
wrapped, so a spare can be
slipped into a pocket. Pack them
in a small zip-lock bag. Extras
will always be gratefully received
by a woman who hasn't yet
experienced the comfort and
convenience.

◆

Jane Vincent-Havelka, over 60,
London, Ontario, Canada

➤ Properly fitted "flight socks" are very effective in preventing deep vein thrombosis or blood clots associated with long haul flights.

➤ Traveling pregnant comes with special risks and considerations. Take advice from your physician well before departure.

➤ Pregnant women need to be careful about what they eat but not all advice you'll receive will be based on scientific evidence!

➤ Women who plan to travel while taking hormones to control fertility or menstrual loss should ensure that they have been using the method for several months before travel. It is best to allow plenty of time for any erratic bleeding or other side effects to settle.

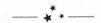

Each night of our five-day canoe trip, we camped on the sandy banks of the Zambezi River or on small islands. Sitting around our campfire one night, a little white village dog appeared with something in his mouth. It was a very large used sanitary towel. He was very difficult to catch and very reluctant to give it up. Those who tried to persuade him were probably risking rabies!

Please dispose of non-biodegradable or slowly biodegradable things properly: either burn them, take them away with you and dispose of them later, or bury them at least two feet deep. And in a snowy environment remember that snow melts, so you need to dig down into soil.

◆

Dr. KS, 30+, physician, Glasgow, UK

➤ It can be hard to find sanitary pads in non-industrialized countries although trying to communicate your requirement to a non-English speaker through charades can be entertaining.

➤ In some regions tampons are not used at all; if these are what you like to use pack plenty.

➤ Be sure to wash hands before inserting a tampon.

➤ Tampons with applicators (like Tampax) are better when water is not readily available for hand washing.

➤ Ziplock or sealable freezer bags are useful for carrying used sanitary items until they can be disposed of properly. Take a good supply.

➤ Menstruating women do not seem to be at increased risk of shark attack when swimming or scuba-diving in the sea.

➤ When one person starts throwing anything other than human waste or toilet paper down a toilet, others copy and then the toilet fills up too quickly with unsuitable waste that should go elsewhere. Try to carry out your sanitary goods if you can. Pads in particular contain uncompostable, non-biodegradable plastics and will be unpleasantly persistent.

Climbing Mount Kenya, I often needed to let my friends, our guide and porters walk on ahead before it was safe to squat unseen. If there was foliage I would throw my used tampon a fair distance only to then find it dangling atop a bush for all to see; I'd then get scratched in the process of recovering the tampon to ditch it further afield but have the same thing happen again! The camp landscape near the summit was lunar. Nowhere to squat unseen, hide my tampon behind or under. Had to wait till it was dark, and was grateful we were leaving before sunrise! I should have packed them out.

♦

Tammy Gillian, 30, veterinary surgeon, Stockport, UK

Chapter 12

CAN IT BE WORMS?
AVOIDING THEM

Travel broadens the mind and loosens the bowels.

—*Anonymous*

I'd been back from India a few months and was sitting on the loo. The long overland trip had left my bowels less reliable and more chaotic than before the trip, but the symptoms were settling. That day though, I was aware of a strange sensation, and looked between my legs to see a worm dangling from my anus. Thankfully it had died of old age. It wasn't moving. My interest in parasitology overcame my revulsion, and I recovered the worm. It was superficially similar to an earthworm, pinkish-white, about twelve inches long: *Ascaris lumbricoides*. This is probably the most common parasite of humans globally. It is a tremendously successful species because its microscopic eggs are incredibly resistant to inhospitable environments; it can blow around in the wind, settle on food, and if you eat this food unwashed or uncooked, this roundworm can set up home inside you. They are utterly revolting but really rather harmless. They have no hooks or suckers and spend their short lives (twelve to eighteen months) sedately swimming upstream within the intestine trying to avoid leaving with your bowel movements. Travelers rarely acquire more than one or two, whereas children of the low-income regions can end up with one hundred or more inside them where they can clog the gut and cause malnutrition or even death. If you pass one, get a stool sample examined under the microscope to see if there are any more, and take treatment if necessary.

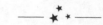

A good medicine for the colic–
Take the hulls of green beans
and distil them and make
water thereof and use that
fasting with a little stale ale
until you are eased thereof.

◆

*Unknown English author,
possibly Dame Juliana
Berners,* circa 1480

Ascaris roundworms and the similar, smaller *Trichuris* whipworms are acquired from contaminated food, but there are a couple of worms that have evolved cleverer means of gaining access to our bodies. First someone with the worms deposits a stool on open ground. There the worm eggs hatch and can penetrate the skin of your feet if you happen to walk barefoot in a contaminated place. They cause a little patch of irritation at the site of penetration and then ride in the bloodstream, eventually setting up home in the gut. Hookworm and *Strongyloides* are the two worms that can enter our bodies by this route. Hookworm rarely colonizes travelers in sufficient numbers to cause symptoms or problems, and infestations will often fade out without people knowing they have carried a few unwelcome hitchhikers. *Strongyloides* can cause some unpleasant illnesses however. Nick Garbutt, wildlife photographer and author, told me about his infestation:

> For the third morning running, I woke up feeling as though my body had been through a mangle—muscles I didn't realize I possessed ached. The cold, damp rainforest floor was to blame. But why did I have technicolor sores covering my feet, the itchy rash around my middle, and dramatic rumblings in my gut? Things got worse when I got home from Madagascar: stomach

rumbles became severe abdominal pain, intestinal volca-
noes erupted frequently, producing farts straight from
Satan's bottom, and life beyond a stone's throw from a
toilet ceased. At the Infectious Disease Unit in Sheffield I
was the center of much interest. "Looks like strongyloi-
diasis," they said and took me up to the lab to look
down the microscope at the culprit: hundreds of them,
Strongyloides stercoralis, microscopic worms that invade
people but are unique among human parasites in being
able to survive in soil for several generations. They bur-
row through the skin of the feet and ride around in the
blood causing irritating rashes. The parasite can then
maintain itself for thirty years without new infections
from the environment. Fortunately, a short course of
horse pills made visits to the loo less frequent, and eating became a pleasure again, although rashes and skin
sores continued for two more months.

The geography worm or *larva migrans* is a different, less
noxious species that causes a very itchy, dry, flaky, red track
usually on the feet or buttocks, wherever the skin has been in
contact with ground contaminated with dog (or cat) feces.
Travelers get it after walking barefoot or sitting on contaminated beaches. The Caribbean and Sri Lanka are two places to
catch it. The dog (or cat) hookworm larva that causes the problem penetrates the skin, then wanders in vain looking for some
dog flesh in which to set up home. It sadly roams the skin for
many weeks, until it finally dies unfulfilled. The head of the
track advances a few millimeters each day; the map-like pattern
it leaves explains why it is also called the geography worm. The
worm will do you no harm, but you will probably want to be
rid of it because of the irritation it causes. Treatment can be by

freezing the head of the worm with liquid carbon dioxide or liquid nitrogen, or with tablets.

Most worms have rather complex life cycles and often spend part of their existence in another species. The tapeworms are perhaps the best known of these, and many people are aware that in less-hygienic environments it is wise to eat any meat well done. Rare steaks can give you beef tapeworm, and rare pork or wild boar steaks may harbor pork tapeworm. The beef tapeworm can reach a length of forty-nine feet yet the symptom that may make you

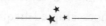

We rented an annex room in Goa. Our toilet (a squatter with a bucket of water to flush it) was fifty yards away. I had dysentery and while making frequent, rushed trips to the bottom of the garden, I wondered how the toilet was kept so clean. One particularly bad day, after many fifty-yard waddles, I found my answer—Todo, the family pig, used toilet offerings as a dietary supplement.

◆

*Ian Carter, 31, the climber,
London, UK*

aware of the presence of a tapeworm is that worm segments that are actually sacks of eggs, come out of the anus. These are mobile and look themselves like tiny worms. This is alarming but is unlikely to harm your health; treatment is straightforward. These life cycles preclude the passing of worms between people. Yet people do worry about this possibility.

Like tapeworms, *Trichinella* are worms that are also acquired from eating inadequately cooked pork, and these are by no means confined to the tropics. If you eat raw or undercooked polar bear, walrus, or wild boar in the Arctic you can acquire trichinosis.

Terrific itching around the anus, especially at night, may also be a sign of a worm infestation. This is the main symptom of threadworm or pinworm. These are tiny and are ubiquitous wherever there are children, both in the industrialized and non-industrialized world. This is the only kind of worm that is commonly passed from person to person. Again, treatment is straightforward, although it is also necessary to combine medical treatment with meticulous personal hygiene, including frequent scrubbing under the fingernails.

The Guinea or Medina worm (*Dracunculus*) is an unpleasant infestation that is caught by swallowing miniscule freshwater "fleas." Drinking only boiled, filtered, or strained water will protect you. It is rapidly nearing extinction throughout much of its range: equatorial Africa, eastern India, Pakistan, southwest Saudi Arabia, and southern Iraq. Don't worry about it.

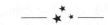

Keeping my balance over the hole in the outhouse in Gansu province (China), I became aware of a movement below. Something was wallowing in the sludge; it had a snout and two eyes. There was a pig living in the toilet pit, guzzling the day's delivery.

◆

Sam Cowan, 27, journalist with wanderlust, Ilford, Essex UK

Tips

➤ Avoid walking barefoot, even on the beach. Wearing shoes helps avoid geography worm, hookworm, as well as injuries from coral and sea urchin spines penetrating the feet.

➤ Excruciating itching around the anus especially at night is likely to be an infestation of threadworm, Enterobius vermicularis. Medicines clear this quickly but be sure while taking treatment that you keep your fingernails cut short and wash meticulously after going to the toilet otherwise you will reinfect yourself and others.

➤ When in less-hygienic environments, steaks and other meats should be freshly cooked and eaten well-done to avoid tapeworms and other gastrointestinal troubles. Meat harboring tapeworm cysts is "measly"—it looks white-speckled.

➤ Beef tapeworm infests not only cows but also buffaloes and yaks, and pork tapeworm can infest dogs.

➤ A selection of unpleasant flukes may be acquired from eating raw or lightly cooked fish and shellfish or water plants (like watercress) which have been contaminated with excrement.

➤ Long-term travelers do not need to take regular courses of worm medicines as some people believe. Most worms do little harm and are usually present in modest numbers.

In two and a half months of cycling alone across China in 1985, I never got sick once, despite always eating at filthy-looking roadside noodle stalls. Meanwhile many travelers who ate in hotels ended up with serious gut problems. I attribute this to the fact that the raw ingredients were cooked in front of me and served within minutes of my order, whereas food in government-run hotels sat around on hot plates for ages. My worst problem was a constantly burned mouth.

◆

Catherine Hopper, 37, cycling Buddhist, Manchester, UK

Fast bowler at the Oval, fresh back in England from an Indian tour, running up to bowl and, suddenly caught short, kept on down the wicket, off the field and into the pavilion—and the lavatory.

◆

Joseph Wilson, 79, retired schoolmaster, Surrey, England

An expatriate mother in Kathmandu asked, "My cook has roundworms. What can I do? Will we all get infested?"

I reassured her. Roundworm eggs need a period of maturation in soil before they become infective so a cook will not pass them on via the food she prepares. The cook was treated and looked healthier and happier subsequently, and the expatriate family stayed worm-free.

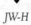

JW-H

Chapter 13

BAD BEASTS
SNAKES AND SPIDERS AND LEECHES, OH MY!

Zookeeper Friedrich Riesfedt dosed his constipated elephant twenty-two times with laxatives as well as feeding him figs and prunes. Finally, while Riesfedt was administering an olive oil enema, the elephant explosively unloaded 200 pounds of excrement, knocked the keeper unconscious and he suffocated beneath the pile.

—*Reported in Himal magazine, Kathmandu, November 1998*

⎯⎯⎯⎯

*B*athrooms and toilets are cool, damp, and often gloomy. Such facilities seem especially attractive refuges for a range of beasts. But what? Is this the place you'll meet spiders, leeches, and venomous snakes? Occasionally an outside loo might harbor a snake, but more likely the animals that surprise you will be smaller: responsible for unnerving scuttling noises and only scary until you find out it was a panicking mouse or fleeing cockroach. Various creatures wander inside searching for pickings, while field wasps and even bees nest in some outside loos. I staggered out one morning up at 11,500 feet in the Helambu region of Nepal. The scene was glorious: frost on the ground; rhododendrons in pink, lilac, and white growing around a dry-stone long-drop. I squatted to perform and noticed large bees dodging my stream of urine; they were coming up to investigate the source of pollution of their nest site. I'd left calmly (flailing about encourages them to attack in force) and the lodge owner persuaded the bees to move house by dropping some flaming rags soaked in kerosene into the pit.

In a simple long-drop you should be able to see any hazardous beasts, but toilet seats might hide something unexpected. In the southern United States, venomous brown spiders (*Loxosceles spp.*) may set up home under the seat of an outside toilet. Occasionally they bite male organs that intrude on the spider's territory. Australian outside lavatories (*dunnies*) carry similar health warnings. Take your flashlight—or better yet, a halogen headlamp—on any nocturnal excursions.

In warm climates in the spring, there are often population explosions of hairy caterpillars; they seem to get everywhere. The "fur" of these animals is actually thousands of minute hypodermics packed with histamines and other irritant chemicals. Check that there are none on the toilet paper before using it, and check your clothes when you get dressed in the morning.

It is astonishing just where small creatures get to. I was running mobile medical clinics in Sri Lanka where mothers complained that when their children defecated, beetles flew out of

I was the first person that morning to use the hole-in-the-ground bush toilet at our campsite in Tarangire National Park, Tanzania. As I started to relieve myself, a very shocked and wet bat flew out of the hole straight into my face.

◆

*Sean Moore, 34,
marketing manager, Northolt,
Middlesex, UK*

Nature called in the middle of the night in India and I crept out to the shack in the courtyard. I was sitting there when—midstream—something cold and wet attacked my private parts. Shrieking I jumped up. I shook as I turned my flashlight toward the toilet. Inside were half a dozen green sucker-footed frogs.

◆

*Margaret Strong,
Exeter, Devon, UK*

the freshly deposited stool. I
didn't believe these tales at first,
but it transpired that certain
dung beetles lay their eggs just
within the anus of small children, the eggs hatch, the beetle
larvae feast lavishly—and harm-
lessly—and then are liberated
when the child "goes."

Groping about in the dark,
or reaching into niches where
you cannot see may be unwise.
A scorpion in Madagascar stung
me when I was rummaging
blindly in the corner of my
rucksack. Scorpions lurk in confined places and are often disturbed by the unwary, and there are dangerous species in
North Africa and the Middle East, Mexico and Arizona, and in
South India; elsewhere their sting is unpleasant but not deadly.
But wherever you are out of doors, use your flashlight at night.
Come evening, tropical toilets and outside bathrooms are often
alive with hungry mosquitoes—this is not a good time for a
visit, unless you have had the forethought to spray the smallest room with insecticide beforehand or have covered yourself
with insect repellent.

Many creatures find both showers and bathrooms attractive.
In a forest reserve in Sri Lanka the only available lights were
hurricane lamps. With the unearthly jungle sounds, the flicker-
ing weird shadows were a little unnerving. I stripped off to
shower when something cold and clammy hit and stuck to my
backside. I jumped, then realized it was only a tree frog confused by the light. The walls were covered in them. They were

On Tioman Island off the east
coast of Malaysia, we had to use
a water-filled squat loo where
lived a gecko. He waited with
his body under the water,
front feet firmly stuck to the
sides of the ceramic pan, head
held high, neck stretched out,
always ready to receive our
humble droppings.

◆

*Mary Kenny, 36, editor
and mother, Delhi, India*

all trying to stay stuck high on the tiled walls, but each was slowly sliding down to the floor. It's strange how, in an unfamiliar environment and especially in poor lighting, the imagination runs riot and even harmless little animals can scare.

There can be surprising finds in latrine pits. When we went to use the open, shallow latrine pit at our base camp in the forest at Ankarana, we often disturbed attractive Madagascar ring-tailed mongooses, *Galidia elegans*. They did not seem so *elegant* when we'd see one emerging from the pit, a half-eaten maggot still protruding from its mouth.

They were responsible for some unnerving nocturnal rustlings on occasion. Pigs and dogs, too, find excreta delicious and in many countries that lack proper sewerage systems, they provide that disposal service.

Wildlife—both large and small—is attracted to our food, and some species can be a terrific nuisance. In some locations ants are an enormous pest. If the sugar is infested, put it into the tea strainer (rather than the cup) and then pour the milk and tea or coffee through the sugar. Thus the ants are sieved from the sugar, leaving an interesting, harmless formic acid piquancy to the beverage. Larger

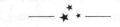

Little red-backed spiders of Australia are said to be venomous and they lurk under toilet seats. When we were in the Outback we were warned to rattle seats before using the toilet.

◆

Barbara Ikin, 47,
Swiss development worker,
Maputo, Mozambique

At George Adamson's camp at Kora National Reserve (Kenya) the toilet was an elephant jawbone. This lower jawbone, when turned upside down, is a perfect toilet seat!

◆

Shailesh Chandaria, 43, tour
operator, Nairobi, Kenya

animal thieves come (theoretically at least) with some increased health risks. Black kites living close to the plush international hotels of Karachi take chicken portions from the hands of guests reclining by the pool, and Sri Lankan hotel crows love snatching beakfuls of sugar from tea trays. Birds can carry salmonella, which might cause gastroenteritis, or at least it might if they leave you anything to eat! And if a dog licks a plate or interferes with your food, you risk *Giardia* and also a nasty parasitic infection called hydatid disease. It is probably best to avoid food that has been shared with birds or larger animals, particularly if they are scavengers by nature.

A notable exception to this, perhaps, is the sought-after Indonesian *kopi luwak*. *Luwak* is the Indonesian for the musk-producing civet cat and *kopi* is coffee. Civets particularly like red coffee berries and swallow down the fruit along with the coffee bean inside. Later the bean is passed in the animal's dung by which time the coffee bean has lost some of its bitterness and is said to be chocolaty, syrupy, earthy, and musty. People willing to harvest the delicacy must be a rare breed since only about 230 kilograms of *kopi lewak* are produced each year in Indonesia, and it comes at a price—around $1,000 a kilogram. Rumor has it that they have the taste for it in Ethiopia, too, so maybe bargain-hunters should start there.

Tips

➤ Nocturnal wanderers in bush or jungle should wear stout shoes and long pants.

➤ It is best to get properly dressed when going for a middle-of-the-night pee in sub-Saharan Africa, or you might contract malaria.

➤ Take a flashlight when seeking relief in the bush or Outback after dark.

➤ Most toilet encounters are with harmless creatures—they're more terrified of you than you need be of them. Pigs or dogs may follow you hoping for something you produce, but these are easily put to flight.

➤ Especially in outside toilets in the tropics, check before you sit or squat. And rattle the seat first.

➤ Just make sure there are no caterpillars or other little meanies on the toilet paper before you use it.

➤ Never put your hand where you cannot see lurking dangers.

➤ A headlamp is very useful when "going" in a dark place; it leaves your hands free for stopping clothes from falling into the mess, etc.

➤ The most dangerous creature that you are likely to encounter in a tropical toilet

At work in Gede, Kenya, the toilet is a long-drop crowned by a box with a seat on it. When flies are disturbed in the depths they try to leave by the only available exit, collide with my bared anatomy, and end up, stunned, in my pants. Strange buzzing sounds sometimes come from below my belt. In Kenya, public toilets are rare, but even when found they may not be the place you want to drop your pants: they are often full of hungry mosquitoes.

Sally Crook, 47, British entomologist and community development advisor, Watamu, Kenya

On the Silk Route between Beijing and Islamabad, taking your trowel into the wilds proved the best toilet. The Chinese lavatories stank—all except one. Here, as each person finished, the local dogs rushed in and ate everything.

♦

Julie Eames, 50, retired salesperson, Southampton, UK

is the mosquito. If you are in a region where mosquito-borne disease is a risk, avoid visits at dusk to primitive
toilets or bathrooms unless you are wearing long clothes
and repellent. Try to time your evening shower for a little
before dusk.

➤ Old World rainforests and also other Asian forests during
the monsoon are places to pick up leeches. They are harmless but revolting, their bites bleed for hours, and these
easily become infected in hot, humid climates. Apply a
DEET-based insect repellent to your ankles or on your shoes
when venturing into leech country. This will keep them off.
Or get them off with a dab of salt or tobacco.

➤ While some travelers rely on alternative remedies, prophy-
laxis, and cures, I would counsel using only conventional
medicines and effective chemical repellents in protecting
yourself from death from malaria. The best repellents are
DEET-based, and those based on natural oils are not effective enough against rampant African malaria-carrying
mosquitoes.

In Kerala, India, I got "the call" and rushed into the forest. Later I felt
something cold on my ankle. Our driver said, "Don't worry, Madam, it
is not dangerous; it is only leech," as he squashed it and my blood oozed
out onto the road. Later still I discovered that my trouser leg was soaked with
blood. Panicking I asked the driver to look away while I disrobed to
investigate. There was only one other bite hole just behind my knee.

◆

Linda Davis, 55, qualified mahout, Haslemere, Surrey, UK

Chapter 14

GOING OUTSIDE
TAKING CARE OF NATURE'S CALL

...when thou wilt ease thyself abroad, thou shalt dig therewith, and
shalt turn back and cover that which cometh from thee.

—*Deuteronomy 23:13*

———

*O*ut in the wilds, enjoying that invigorating feeling of being away from people, you take a deep breath and that smell reaches your nostrils; that smell or a vision of a brown deposit—or worse—the realization you've just stepped in it. It just spoils your moment, your day. But maybe the poor unfortunate who left the deposit had nowhere else to "go." It's a problem, isn't it? Or is it? Actually it is not so difficult to dispose of your offerings responsibly. Ideally your turd should be buried in the top six to eight inches of organic soil, and covered with six inches of dirt; in this way your crap will be hygienically and efficiently absorbed into the nutrient cycle, and it is buried deep enough to discourage retrieval by scavengers. Animals may investigate deposits that are left above ground or shallowly buried, some will eat it, and badgers and dogs even like rolling in the stuff. A trowel or ice ax will assist you in conscientious burial. Hikers who are caught short might try using their boot heel to excavate a hole, but this will only work where the ground is soft and loamy. Then, bowels moved, you can burn the toilet paper (but beware of causing a forest fire) and then cover it well with dirt and leaf litter and tamp it down. Contact with soil and leaf litter speeds decomposition. Kathleen Meyer, author of *How* *to Shit in the Woods*, suggests stirring dirt into your turd with a stick before covering it. You could pick up a rock, crap, then replace the rock, but the next person might get an unpleasant surprise if they try the same trick, and actually squashing excrement under a rock slows nature's disposal system. Why not use a rock to excavate a latrine hole? Or better still, make sure you "go" in the morning before leaving your campsite, where facilities may be provided or are easier to improvise.

In some parts of North America, walkers and climbers are encouraged, and sometimes required, to carry out all their

On our way to a new clinic, I needed a pee and asked the driver to stop. I walked off toward a small group of trees to hide behind them. Suddenly my Cambodian colleague came running after me waving his arms. "You can't go there! That's just the kind of place for a land mine." What could I do? Bouff! I just pulled down my pants and pissed on the road. Everyone could see but I didn't care. What else could I do?

◆

Veronique McConnell, 37, nurse just after the war in Cambodia, France

excrement from a wilderness area. Lack of suitable containers, biodegradable bags, and disposal facilities in Europe make this option unattractive but dog owners dispose of canine crap so why shouldn't we pack ours out, too? No one thinks of doing it but it is standard on certain military exercises and surely it is the only way on our increasingly overcrowded planet? Otherwise burial is the recommended method. If in snow, dig down to soil. When the ground is frozen, Meyer suggests packing it out. With regard to a popular extreme technique for backcountry disposal, "frosting a rock," Meyer cautions employing it only in the most remote and open locations (sunny exposures above timberline or desert regions), where other hikers do not abound and rain storms are not on the horizon. With a stone, trowel your deposit into a half-inch coating—like frosting (icing) a cake—across the surface of a sun-facing rock. Spreading thinly speeds and assists the natural breakdown when excrement is exposed to direct sunlight, as ultraviolet rays and also the drying process inactivate nasty microbes. But beware of contaminating very fragile ecosystems. This option may seem rather unaesthetic, yet dealing with your own products is so much better than being faced with someone else's and is far preferable to the selfish drop-and-run technique practiced by so many. This is particularly noticeable in the Himalayas where my children have imported others' excreta into our tent!

Remember that a stream may be someone else's water supply so never "go" into water, but defecate at least fifty yards from any streams and rivers, and downstream of any settlement. When camping, take your own

There's nothing like sphagnum moss for a clean and dry wipe. Green leaves aren't too bad and grass works if the blades are long and you have enough of it. But for a really jobby experience go for sphagnum. It's better than a bidet. The Highlands of Scotland are carpeted in the stuff. Grab a clump and wipe the worst off with a wet handful. Squeeze the water out of another pile and you have a towel for the perfect wipe experience, unless of course the midges are out. Then you will pay with bitten balls and bum.

◆

James Carnegie, 36,
mountaineer and Highland
bagpiper, Cambridge, UK

In rural north India, people will say that they are going to the maidan—literally an open space or field—when they need to go for a shit.

◆

Rajendra S. Khadka, editor of
Travelers' Tales Nepal

drinking water from above your site and defecate downhill. Although urine is less harmful than stools, try to be responsible about where you pee, too. Avoid urinating at the foot of crags, in cave entrances, or behind buildings. And "go" at least 50 yards from paths and 200 yards from climbing huts, refuges, or other buildings.

When traveling by vehicle, there is often less choice in where we can excrete. Taking the bus from Antananarivo to Fort Dauphin in Madagascar, I joined a line of women squatting behind a wall, a trickle of urine emerging from beneath the skirt of each of us. We stayed the night in a very basic *hotely*; the toilet there was a choice of a rather overfull slop bucket on the balcony overlooking the main street, a squat toilet which was blocked and seething with maggots, or "the bush." My flashlight was unreliable, and

Running a temporary clinic in western Madagascar, we resorted to using the cotton fields as a latrine. But although we always tried to wait until darkness fell, our bottoms shone like beacons in the moonlight. Here was another disadvantage of being white: our Malagasy colleagues could "go" unobserved.

◆

Dr. Anne Denning, 37, ophthalmic surgeon, Bournemouth, UK

A headlamp is especially useful when relieving oneself in unusual places, much easier than gripping a flashlight in one's teeth—just turn it off before exposing oneself.

◆

Jean Sinclair, 33, nurse, biologist, and expeditionary, Cambridge, UK

the "bush" comprised unpleasant, spiky thorn bushes so I was relieved to be able to teeter over the slop bucket in the privacy of darkness. I wonder whose job it was to empty the bucket in the morning. The contents can be useful. In the Hebrides a hundred years ago, chamber pots were emptied into a communal storage barrel so that Harris tweed could be soaked in urine to condition the cloth.

Going outside for relief can have its hazards, even for locals. In India, space is at such a premium that the roadside is one of the few places people can squat. They venture out after dark and are hit by speeding cars. In Nepal, women are rendered night-blind by poor nutrition and the demands of pregnancy. Thus pregnant women there have almost double the risk of accidental death than nonpregnant women, because they often fall off some dangerous ledge while out after dark opening their bowels. It is worth trying to avoid those unscheduled night calls, and if you do need to go outside make sure you carry a good functioning flashlight or headlamp.

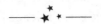

My bladder was about to burst. Three of us were wedged into a second floor room with the only exit a creaky door just beyond my snoring companions. Past that was a precipitous staircase to the room where four generations of the family were sleeping, and beyond them lay doors bolted for the night. It was pitch-dark and I knew I'd never make it outside without waking the entire household and possibly killing myself in a tumble. My only recourse was the window by my cot that opened to the tile roof. I peed a torrent into the Himalayan night and have never felt such relief, realizing only afterward that someone may have been sleeping on the porch below.

◆

Larry Habegger, 53, writer and editor, San Francisco, California

For females, expeditionary Jean Sinclair adds, a wide mouthed tin, such as Mornflakes porridge oats, which comes with a plastic lid, works well, provided you have been very skillful with your can opener to produce a smooth edge. If women want to keep clear of a messy toilet, have difficulties squatting over a squatty or can't hover over an airline toilet during turbulence, they may want to invest in a Shewee (www.shewee.com) or Pstyle (www.thepstyle.com), devices that allow women to pee standing.

Many predators, including snakes, scorpions, and giant centipedes, are nocturnal and you could encounter one in your nighttime perambulations. They also have the unfortunate habit of curling up in shoes and clothing and get upset when you, the owner, attempt to get dressed before a nocturnal outing. Check before you dress then and put on stout shoes and long pants to help protect you from these creatures. Be aware though, that few animals want to fight, so if you don't creep up on them but announce your arrival by stomping clumsily

When relieving yourself in the Antarctic always check that what you intended to leave outside the suit is actually left out-side the suit. The hood can harvest that which you didn't want to collect.

♦

Russ Ladkin, 39, Antarctic meteorological instrument engineer, Cambridge, UK

Smart male trekkers in Nepal sleep with an empty plastic jar with a wide mouth. If the need arises at night, they piss into the jar and thereby avoid unwanted nocturnal encounters.

♦

Rajendra S. Khadka, editor of Travelers' Tales Nepal

and noisily, you will be most unlikely to meet anything nasty. The light makes you visible as well as allowing you to sidestep hazards of the night.

Some years ago my husband took me on a miserable trek in the monsoon rains. At the road head in East Nepal, we found spaces in a squalid second floor dormitory. I'd forgotten to pack a flashlight and the cheap local light wasn't working. The lodge provided candles and matches though. I needed a pee in the night. It was wet and windy so the candle went out several times as I scrambled down the steep outside steps to the toilet shack. I managed my pee by lighting more matches, but as I headed back inside, a drunk pissed off the balcony all over me. If only my flashlight had been working.

Several women travelers have told me that they reduce the amount that they drink if there are no "civilized" toilets available so that they don't *need* to pass water as often. I can understand the reasoning behind this but, especially in the hot climates, this is a dangerous strategy. Reducing fluid intake will increase the chances of heat stroke and urinary tract infections; it may also lead to kidney stones. Everyone needs to produce three good volume urinations a day, toilet or no toilet.

A collective calculation of the amount of excreta that open defecation adds to the environment is an interesting, participatory method of helping communities to realize the magnitude and extent of their sanitation problem. Villagers estimate the amount of feces one person produces in a day, then multiply to calculate contribution per family, per week, per year, and so forth. In Mosmoil, Bangladesh the community calculated that 50,000 tons of human excreta were being added to their village environment every year. Flow diagrams are then drawn to trace contamination routes to ponds, household utensils and, most importantly, to food through hands, flies, chickens, etc.

◆

Andy Robinson, 38, water and sanitation specialist, St-Bon-Courchevel, France

Tips

➤ When hiking in toilet-free zones, check what you are expected to do with your excreta; some North American parks provide trowels or suitable bags as well as disposal sites.

➤ In shared sleeping accom-
modation, you won't want to
disturb others when you get
up to pee. If you keep one
eye closed when you turn on
the light in the bathroom,
your night vision will be
preserved in that eye and
you will be able to navigate
back to bed in almost total
darkness by opening that
closed eye.

➤ Composting dry toilets have
been built in a few remote
locations. Carefully follow
the instructions on how to
use it so that it continues to
function and remains smell-
free after your visit.

➤ Remember that in many
resource-poor regions people
"go" at night; the dark offers
privacy so if there are no
facilities follow suit, but
make sure you take a reliable
flashlight. The light will help
you avoid treading in others'
deposits, and you can check
the location for safety, too.

I needed a shit in the middle of
the night at our forest base camp
at Ankarana, Madagascar. As I
walked back, my feeble penlight
stopped working and I was lost.
I didn't have much on so I was
loath to shout for help. I was
just contemplating waiting for
four hours until dawn broke,
when Jean-Elie let out an enormous snore to guide me safely
back to my hammock.

◆

*Dr. Anne Denning, 37, ophthal-
mic surgeon, Bournemouth, UK*

Beware of what you squat over,
especially at night: I have been
unpleasantly surprised by fire
ants in Bali, by thistles and
stinging nettles in Ireland, and
by sand fleas in Peru.

◆

*Anne Peniston, 46, international
public health worker, Nepal*

➤ If there are no en suite toilet facilities or the electricity supply is unreliable, make sure your flashlight is handy when you settle down to sleep for the night. Otherwise you might have trouble locating the loo later.

➤ When walking into the bush or jungle for relief, wear stout shoes and long pants; this will protect you from scorpion stings and snake-bite as well as thorn scratches and stubbed toes.

➤ Get dressed when you venture outside for relief after dark. If you have an accident or bump into someone, you will avoid embarrassment, and it also should reduce the chances of being bitten by mosquitoes.

➤ When "going" outside and you think others are around, whistling or singing will warn people of your whereabouts; in Asia the locals will understand—they may think you are scared of ghosts.

On a six-month overland tour of Africa we were told we must burn all used toilet paper. After a few drinks, Lucie visited the toilet tent. As the rest of us relaxed under the stars, there was a loud explosion and we turned to see the toilet tent in flames. Lucie, in setting fire to her toilet paper had ignited methane gas. She was all right but in her panic had left her pants in the inferno.

◆

Anthea Iva, 28, adventure travel consultant, Victoria, Australia

In rural Bangladesh, there are millions of people, little cover, and locals find foreigners fascinating. It is impossible, therefore, for women to relieve themselves outdoors in privacy. We traveled with three large cheap black Chinese umbrellas to hide behind when I needed to go.

◆

Barbara Ikin, 47, development adviser, Mozmbique

➤ Rustlings and scuttlings
sound louder at night; shin-
ing your flashlight toward
some nocturnal monster will
reveal a chicken, cat, mouse,
or some-such small harmless
wanderer.

➤ In some regions you may
encounter half-wild dogs; if
they threaten you, stoop
down as if to pick up a
stone. This will put most
dogs to flight. Carrying a
stout walking stick is an additional protection against village or street dogs.

> ── ⁎ ⁎ ⁎ ──
>
> When "going" outside in the
> Antarctic, excavate a hole and
> then sit on the spade for a com-
> fortable shit, but beware, at sub-
> zero temperatures you will stick
> to a metal handle. Choose a
> wooden-handled spade.
>
> ◆
>
> *Steve Colwell, 32, meteorologist,*
> *British Antarctic Survey,*
> *Cambridge, UK*

➤ Burning used toilet paper will reduce pollution and
unsightly litter. Most responsible travelers will burn that
which will burn and then bury everything. Methane gas is
explosive, but this should only be a risk in confined, unven-
tilated spaces.

➤ Don't "hang on" to bladder or bowel contents longer than
feels comfortable, and don't restrict the amount you drink
in order to avoid peeing; these are unhealthy practices.

➤ If women want to keep clear of a messy toilet, have difficulties squatting over a squatty, or can't hover over an airline
toilet during turbulence, they may want to invest in a washable Shewee or Pstyle.

➤ At high altitude, temperatures plummet at night and going outside for a pee is a chilling experience. It can also be hazardous since you may slip on ice even inside the toilet.

➤ Some trekkers and mountaineers take acetazolamide (Diamox) capsules to speed acclimatization and reduce high-altitude insomnia; this medicine is a mild diuretic (it increases urine production) so take them in the morning otherwise you will be awakened by your bladder in the night.

➤ Reindeer have a passion for human urine and so are easily tamed, ridden, and harnessed: watch where you pee in Lapland!

➤ When relieving yourself outdoors, think beyond preserving your modesty and avoid places where others might want to loiter or rest. Bury your excreta six inches (15cm) deep if you can.

Middle of the Bering Strait, heaving seas, strong winds, and icebergs, ten hours out from Cape Prince of Wales, paddling single-seat kayaks. The toilet procedure was for two people to raft together. Robert then held my kayak while I unzipped my dry suit and carefully pushed a beaker down between my legs. Started to pee and when my thumb became warm I knew it was about to overflow. Now the tricky bit of extracting the beaker through a very tight dry suit without spilling it, trusting Robert not to let the kayak go.

◆

Trevor Potts, 49, adventurer, Argyll, Scotland

Chapter 15

BATHING
HAZARDS AND TECHNIQUES IN
UNUSUAL CIRCUMSTANCES

Wading in, as the hanging mist over the river began to
lighten and lift.... I swam a little way off, into an upstream
eddy by the bank, and there, luckily, all alone I learned the
most important lesson for tranquil conduct of life in the
jungle: never, ever, shit in a whirlpool.

—*Redmond O'Hanlon, Into the Heart of Borneo*

━━━

*H*ow safe is bathing outdoors? It is hard to imagine
anything more appealing and natural than soaking in
some warm, natural body of water somewhere. But is
it risky? I've swum in a wonderfully private subterranean river
in Madagascar. I've bathed in fast-moving Amazonian waters
but, with all the tales I'd heard about piranhas, I was on edge
and when toothless fish came nibbling at my stomach, my
imagination invented man-eating beasts. It seems to have been
the hyperbolic accounts published by Theodore Roosevelt that
are the basis of the fearsome reputation of the piranha: there
are no reliable accounts of human deaths due to these fish.
Authenticated accounts are also wanting of damage done by the
mysterious candiru fish that is said to lodge itself inside swimmers' urethras. Travelers' folklore has it that if the victim is
male, the only treatment is penile amputation. In fact, the fish
does not seem to be so misanthropic. The candiru is a parasite
that prefers to settle down inside the gills of other fish.

The biggest real threat from freshwater bathing is drowning— or losing the soap. There are a few nasty aquatic animals that may cause some grief but the chances of meeting any are slim. The reputations of many "dangerous" beasts seem exaggerated, although tropical South American rivers can harbor stingrays which can cause exceedingly nasty injuries. In Africa, crocodiles and hippos are dangerous. There is a river in western Madagascar called Tsiribihina that means, "Where you mustn't swim." Why? Because Nile crocodiles will probably eat you. Take local advice before bathing outdoors.

The risks of upsetting a large animal are small, yet there are some real hazards. Bathing outdoors in much of Africa can put you at risk of schistosomiasis (also known as bilharzia). This parasite spends part of its life in freshwater snails and part in larger animals such as humans. People suffering from bilharzia pass eggs in their urine or feces, and if these enter suitable, well-oxygenated freshwater, they will hatch out and swim off in search of a snail to infest. Here the parasite multiplies then goes

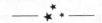

In the Apo Kayan, far in the north of East Kalimantan, villagers had delineated three sections of the river for different uses. The most upstream section was for fetching drinking water, next there was the bathing and washing area, while the section farthest downstream was for defecating. There is an art to crapping in the river. Wear a sarong rather than shorts or skirt and underwear. Firstly, move in far enough from the bank where the water is actually flowing (near the bank it is often very slow moving indeed) or you will find yourself using your hands to stir up the water to get your turd to travel away. Secondly, face upstream. It is disconcerting to be confronted with one's own emission as it flows past.

◆

Glenys Chandler, Ph.D., 55, community development specialist, Melbourne, Australia

out into a free-swimming stage again, but in this form the miniscule worm is capable of digesting its way through the flesh of anyone who happens to be paddling or bathing. This causes "swimmers' itch" as the worm penetrates the skin and then the parasite rides in the bloodstream until eventually it sets up home in bladder (*Schistosoma haematobium*) or bowel (*Schistosoma mansoni*), where it settles down to producing millions of eggs. Travelers are infected when swimming, paddling, or even showering in waters contaminated with human waste, which usually means that the victim has paddled or swum within

It took years of traveling to develop an efficient laundry technique. Try this. Keep your clothes on in the shower. Get soaked. Turn off the shower. Then rub yourself (and your clothes) all over with soap. You can then either continue showering to rinse the clothes before taking them off, wringing them out, and hanging them to dry or you can remove them for an extra-thorough rub under the shower to get rid of those nasty stains and smells.

◆

James Carnegie, 36, aspiring travel writer, Cambridge, UK

200 yards of a village or point where people use water—for washing clothes perhaps, or where village children romp. Infected travelers tend to get ill with a fever, and once alerted to this infection, there is a very effective cure in the drug praziquantel. A blood test done *more* than six weeks after last possible exposure to the parasite will establish the diagnosis. The highest-risk geographical regions are the great lakes of the east African Rift Valley, but the infection can be acquired from many freshwater lakes, streams, and slow-moving rivers where there is waterweed for the snails to feed on. There are foci in the Middle East, and in the tropical Americas (northeast Brazil, the Guianas, Surinam, Venezuela, and some Caribbean islands).

The species that occur in Africa and the Middle East (*Schistosoma haematobium* and *S. mansoni*) and America (*Schistosoma mansoni*) are slow penetrators. Since it takes at least ten minutes to get through the skin, a quick splash across a suspect stream should do you no harm; vigorous towelling dry after bathing also kills any parasites caught in the act of skin penetration. Unfortunately Oriental schistosomiasis, *Schistosoma japonicum*, which occurs in parts of China, Taiwan, Vietnam, the Philippines, and two remote valleys in central Sulawesi, penetrates within a few minutes and is altogether a much nastier parasite.

➤ When in bilharzia country, avoid bathing or paddling on shores within 200 meters of African villages or places where people use the water a great deal, especially reedy shores or where there is a lot of waterweed.

➤ Bathing and swimming early in the morning carries a

Baring your bum to the dark depths of a tropical long-drop, or braving an ice-cold al fresco waterfall shower may be a challenge to the toughest traveler. Being paralyzed from the shoulders down adds a whole new dimension.

I've cut an appropriately placed hole in the wheelchair, and using single-sided sticky tape and insulating foam I've made a comfortable toilet seat. The product is caught and wrapped in newspaper, which is available and cheap everywhere from Timbuktu to Kathmandu, and it is compostable.

Where showers aren't wheelchair-accessible, I do the sweaty sponge bath in bed routine. However, more than a week of this "pushing the dirt around" isn't socially acceptable so eventually I resort to having buckets of water thrown over me outdoors. I try to find somewhere private, otherwise end up being surrounded by hysterical local children.

◆

Gordon Rattray, 34, Scotsman living in Belgium, author of Access Africa: safaris for people with limited mobility.

lesser risk for bilharzia than bathing in the last half of
the day.

➤ If bathing, swimming, paddling, or wading in freshwater
that you think may be risky, try to get out of the water
within ten minutes. Then dry off thoroughly and vigorously
with a towel; this will kill any parasites on their way in
through your skin.

➤ If your bathing water comes from a source that may be contaminated with bilharzia, try to ensure that the water is
taken from the lake in the early morning and stored snail-
free, otherwise it should be filtered or have Dettol or
Cresol added.

➤ Bathing early in the morning carries a lesser risk for bilharzia than bathing in the last half of the day.

➤ If you have been exposed to bilharzia parasites, arrange a
screening blood test more than six weeks since your last
contact with suspect water.

➤ Bilharzia is never acquired from sea bathing.

There is another hazard of tropical rivers and bathing in
them; this is onchocerciasis or river blindness. This is a problem in much of tropical sub-Saharan Africa between 19°N and
17°S, and it also occurs in parts of Central and tropical South
America. This unpleasant worm is transmitted near fast-flowing
rivers through the bites of small biting blackflies, *Simulium
damnosum*. These pestilential flies are a nuisance even in
regions (like Asia) where river blindness is absent. Sand-fly
bites cause big, very itchy lumps in the skin, often with a
bloody speck at the center. River blindness has a variety of

manifestations, since it invades many parts of the body, but in travelers and expatriates the worms most commonly make the skin incredibly itchy, and the itching is usually confined to a single limb or only the arms or just the legs. People need to have had extremely heavy infestations for many years before the eyes are threatened. Keep these daytime biters off with long loose clothes and a DEET-based insect repellent applied to any exposed skin.

If you want to bathe outdoors and there are lots of people about, it is possible to bathe modestly by putting on a sarong or lungi. This is a tube of cotton cloth that is wide enough to cover all essentials so that you can bathe comprehensively but modestly under a village water-spout in full view. For women, a long wraparound skirt can be used in the same way. Such garments will dry quickly in the midday sun along with your freshly washed underwear.

Bathing indoors has some advantages. In Indonesia each bathroom has a *bak mandi*, a water tank used to wash the bottom after using the toilet, flush the toilet, and also for bathing. The all-purpose technique is to scoop from the *bak mandi*. It is not a bath to climb into. Travelers often upset their Indonesian hosts by washing in the *bak mandi*, thereby polluting it and making it necessary to empty and clean the whole thing. In much of Southeast Asia there are similar cool water tanks. Water taken straight from a

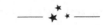

To avoid flooding a Vietnamese bathroom, check the wash basin. In the absence of a waste pipe, take the bucket from beside the loo, and place it under the basin before washing. You will need the contents for flushing the loo—but remember to reposition the bucket beneath the basin before washing again; it's easy to forget.

♦

Angela Rowe, 49, musician/IT worker, Swansea Valley, Wales

sun-baked tank on the roof would scald the bather, so often it is stored in huge terracotta pots inside the bathroom.

When I was about fourteen years old, I went to Paris on a school trip. We stayed in a cheap hotel, and the double room that Anne and I shared contained two beds and— behind a skimpy curtain—a toilet, wash basin, and a useful little footbath. We thought this was marvelously civilized; we'd spend our summer days tramping around the hot city and come back grubby and footsore, when there was usually a queue for the shower. Our teacher laughed when he heard us enthuse about the footbath. "It's a *bidet* not a footbath! It's for washing your bottom after you've used the lavatory...."

In English-speaking countries, taps are often labeled with a C for cold and H for hot. In France, *chaud* is hot, so hot taps have C on them. In Spain too a C indicates the hot tap. In Portugal, they are labeled Q (*quente*) for hot and F (*frio*) for the cold water taps. In some places hot taps have a red dot on them

Having a good wash can demand some subtlety, but cleaning wonders can be achieved, in the privacy of a very small tent, by squatting over a small dish of water and using a cloth, soap, and preferably a close friend to scour your back. Start before sunset (with its attendant frost or mosquitoes) and begin at the savory end of your person, the lips. Then systematically work your way down. If you wish to use the cloth ever again, keep green ones for the upper part of your lovely body, and blue for bottoms. Finally hang the cloths out to dry, which they do even in a heavy frost at night, and once dry (usually about an hour after dawn), you can pack them into separate polyethylene bags. When they begin to get a bit fruity, just burn them and use new ones.

◆

Dr. Jim Waddell, 66, retired consultant internal physician, Cirencester, UK

and cold is indicated by blue, but in much of Asia the plumber seems to have set out to tease his clients by connecting pipes the other way around. Labels on doors can be confusing, too. I opened a door on a Portuguese railway train that was marked *Lavatório* (and, helpfully there was a French translation *Toilette,*

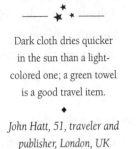

Dark cloth dries quicker in the sun than a light-colored one; a green towel is a good travel item.

◆

John Hatt, 51, traveler and publisher, London, UK

too). Inside I found a wash hand basin. The loo was behind a door marked WC. In Spain the toilets are called *Los Servicios.*

At high altitude, daytime sunshine can be warming but temperatures plummet after dark in the mountains. A toothbrush left soaking in water overnight in the high Andes or Himalayas will be encased in a block of ice by morning. In these kinds of climates you may not want to do much washing at all, and there is sense in developing a technique for minimal hygiene. And if you decide to wash your hair, you risk it freezing on the head. You do however need to apply plenty of moisturizers and also sunscreen to stop you turning into a prune.

Tips

➤ Make sure you wash your hands with soap and water after visiting any public toilet and before eating: your

I went to shower in the make-shift cubicle under a tree, in the remote Luangwa Valley, Zambia. There was a snake curled up inside: thick, grayish, about a yard long. It left through the reed wall as swiftly as I left through the space that acted as the door.

◆

Chris McIntyre, 33, guidebook author, tour operator, and safari addict, London, UK

microbes won't harm you but other peoples' will. Attention to personal hygiene is more important when traveling than it is at home.

➤ In regions where people cannot afford sanitation, there are more flies and microbes about so any scratches or wounds need to be thoroughly cleaned.

➤ Keeping your fingernails cut short will make them easier to keep clean. The speed that fingernails (and hair) grow depends upon environ-mental temperatures. Adventur-ers in the Arctic and Antarc-tic may not need to cut their nails for many months, while in the tropics they seem to need cutting every few days. Pack some nail clippers if traveling to warm climates.

➤ Malaria mosquitoes love the smell of sweaty feet, so a shower before dusk will reduce the bite rate. However avoid using highly perfumed cosmetics—they are attracted to pleasant scents too.

➤ Take local advice before bathing outdoors.

➤ One of the most dangerous animals in tropical Africa is the hippopotamus. They come out of the rivers to graze at dusk

---

——— ✱ * ———

I asked, in Calcutta, for the bathroom and was ushered into a room that was absolutely bare, apart from the concrete floor and a bucket of water. "But I wanted the loo, not a bath." I said. My hostess took me back into the room and pointed to a small hole in the wall and a long straw brush. Yes, one crapped on the floor and then had to brush the turds out into the hole with the brush, using the bucket of water to lubricate the process as well as wash the hands (and the bottom of course), or even take a shower.

◆

Alan Smith, Australian develop-ment worker, Myanmar

and during overcast days, so
beware if you are bathing in
the river or strolling along
the riverbank. If you disturb
them and are between
them and the river—their
refuge—they may flatten you
in their panic to get back
into the water.

➤ In sub-Saharan Africa if you
are on the riverbank you
may be on the menu. Watch
out for Nile crocodiles. They
eat about a thousand Afri-
cans a year.

➤ Glance around on entering
outside shower cubicles;

Convenient bathing machines
are kept on the beach attended
by strong and careful persons,
affording the temptation of
bathing in the sea without possibility of observation. These con-
sist of a commodious wooden
chamber…floored with open
boards, in which firmly secured
to the framework of the
machine, the most timid bather
may enjoy the sea without
apprehension or molestation.

◆

*Robert Wake, Southwold
and Its Vicinity (1839)*

they may be already occupied. Wet broken glass is also difficult to see—until you stand on it.

➤ Avoid stepping on stingrays, when bathing or wading in
South American rivers, by shuffling along in the water; this
disturbs these fish, and they will swim away before you
inadvertently step on them.

➤ Never dive headfirst into unknown waters, especially if
turbid. It is always safer to jump in feet first.

➤ Plan where you will put the soap when bathing in rivers,
otherwise it is likely to float off downstream and away out
of reach.

➤ A large, tough plastic bag is useful for soaking dirty clothes overnight so that they are then easy to wash. Your hotel sink may have no plug, and improvised stoppers will not maintain a full sink all night.

During the COVID-19 pandemic we encouraged our pupils to wash their hands for as long as it took to sing Happy Birthday—twice. Whenever I walked past the toilets I could hear joyous little voices singing the birthday song.

♦

Anna Liisa Griffin, primary teacher, Kathmandu, Nepal

➤ T-shirts and jeans are not good travelers' clothes. They are slow to dry after they've been washed and they are not cool to wear in hot climates.

➤ If you need to get your underwear to dry quickly, roll it in a hotel towel.

➤ In Southeast Asia, scoop bathing water onto you from the water tank; don't climb into it or rinse your feet in it or you will upset the locals.

➤ If using an outside bathroom in the tropics, you may wish to avoid bathing around 6 P.M. when mosquitoes are at their hungriest; it is best to shower just before they gather at dusk.

➤ If you are renting a cheap hotel room that boasts en suite facilities, step into the bathroom—before the room boy leaves—to check for smells and listen awhile for drips. Water music from leaking plumbing can cause insomnia, and the smells from some facilities can be so overpowering as to make you wish they weren't en suite.

➤ Wash basins in cheap hotels often lack a plug. Universal sink plugs are available, otherwise half a squash ball or half a lime work well. As a last resort, a scrumpled bit of plastic shopping bag will suffice.

➤ Observe good hygiene etiquette and sneeze into your elbow. This reduces transmission of colds and more serious respiratory infections.

➤ During the COVID-19 pandemic the World Health Organization recommended that people should frequently wash their hands with soap and water for as long as it takes to sing the Happy Birthday song twice or—if there is no soap and water and the hands look clean—rub in alcohol hand sanitizing gel (60% or more) for 20–30 seconds.

➤ Muslims in Pakistan say that couples should purify themselves after love-making by having a "full bath" including washing their hair. People who walk out with wet hair after taking a shower therefore provoke giggles.

The guest house in Darjeeling had no hot water, and the autumn chill that hung over the Himalayan foothills discouraged anything more than a wash-cloth bath, but for some reason just shy of masochism I decided to take a "shower" the way the locals did, by dipping a bucket into a cistern and pouring water over my head. The first bucket was bone chilling, but after that shock I hardly felt the rest, and at the end of a good scrubbing every nerve ending danced. I was so invigorated the day took on a new crispness, and I repeated the ritual every day for a week. That first bucket never felt good, but after bathing I felt alive in ways no other kick-start could accomplish.

◆

Larry Habegger, 53, writer and editor, San Francisco, California

Chapter 16

CHILDREN
KEEPING LITTLE ONES HEALTHY

There's a rumble in your tum,
That makes you feel glum,
Diarrhea,
Diarrhea.

There's a feeling in your rear,
That fills you full of fear,
Diarrhea,
Diarrhea.

Then it comes out of your bum,
Like a bullet from a gun,
Diarrhea,
Diarrhea.

—*Discovered and remastered by Max Tew and Seb Howarth, 10, Cambridge, UK*

———

*C*hildren are adaptable animals but unfamiliar lavatories can intimidate them: children's fertile imaginations can make all manner of things lurk in the shadows within. A good, powerful flashlight might persuade a reluctant child into a dark toilet, but even so, once inside, many children will be scared of falling into the hole of a squat toilet. When my oldest son was three, we went to live in a village on an island in the middle of Nepal's biggest river. He was intimidated by our outside squat toilet and coped by perfecting the technique of peeing into it from outside the door, or using a potty. When he needed to open his bowels, he and I squatted together. He'd squat over the hole with me behind him for support. He still gave many a backward glance at the intimidating chasm beneath his bum.

Even as children grow older and bolder, the squatty can just be too large for a child to squat over; they need more help than with a pedestal WC—and "training seats" are useless. A potty thus might be handy even if, under normal circumstances, the child has outgrown one; they are useful if the child can't manage to squat or if the toilet is a long, dark walk outside.

Disposable diapers are a tre-

—— ★* * ——

In much of Asia, toddlers don't use diapers, but run around bare-bottomed; when they do "perform" there is usually a dog around to lick the child clean. If there's no dog then there are other resources: I once saw an older brother wiping a younger's bottom with a rock.

◆

Brian Peniston, 47, international conservation and development worker, Nepal

mendous boon to parents because they absorb so much more than terry-cloth diapers, but they can be very expensive if purchased in resource-poor countries: they are usually at least twice the price they are at home. And disposal is a problem. I have tried burning them, pouring on kerosene and igniting them, and even wondered whether the solution was to wrap them around some Semtex explosive—they are indestructible. The only eco-sensitive action is to try to avoid using disposables. If you have soiled disposable diapers, pack them out and find somewhere to discard them later. This option will be more tolerable if the poop is first deposited in the nearest toilet. Otherwise, and as an absolute last resort, you might simply have to bury them, deep. Putting them into the hotel garbage will often result in them being dumped somewhere where dogs will play with them, and they'll end up blowing around the streets.

Consider using at least some cloth diapers; cleaning of the diaper is made easier and less unpleasant if disposable liners are

used since these can be dropped
into a pit latrine or flushed away
with the poop. Be aware that
these liners are robust, they
readily block simple flush toilets
and they do not compost. Be
sensitive, therefore, about where
you dispose of these, too. Families who are staying in one place
for a few days will be able to
wash cloth diapers, and one way

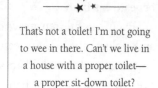

That's not a toilet! I'm not going
to wee in there. Can't we live in
a house with a proper toilet—
a proper sit-down toilet?

◆

Alexander Howarth, 3,
on arriving in his new home
in rural Nepal

to detoxify a soiled diaper is to soak it in diluted liquid bleach
before washing. Bleach is readily available in a surprising
number of quite remote destinations, so it is not necessary to
bring soaking solution from home. It is risky stuff to have in
your luggage and it is heavy, yet it will be inexpensive when
bought abroad.

The risk of intestinal problems is great in travelers, particularly in regions with fewer resources than at home. The risks to
traveling children are even greater, since they love exploring
unhygienic places and they also have less immunity than
adults. Some cautious physicians would even suggest that children under three years of age should not travel to areas where
filth-to-mouth disease is rife. The highest-risk regions are probably tropical Latin America and the Indian subcontinent,
including Nepal, where traveling small children will have a
greater than 50–50 chance of getting some fairly unpleasant
form of diarrhea or dysentery, and they also risk other filth-to-
mouth diseases including typhoid and hepatitis A.

The little ones need to be fully immunized before travel;
immunization is actually more important in traveling families
than those who stay at home. In countries (like the U.S.) where
there is a successful immunization program, there is a low risk

of contracting infectious disease, because there are few susceptible people around to pass these infections on. In many resource-poor countries immunization coverage may be only 20 to 50 percent and so the pool of possible infectors is great.

We were on holiday in Thailand, recuperating from a simpler life in Nepal, where the meat was tough and so rice and lentils were our usual fare. My two-year-old's eyes lit upon the rubbery chicken sausages on display on the breakfast buffet. He devoured eight with gusto. At about 2 A.M. he awoke distressed and crying. He was disoriented and scared, trying to escape the snakes that he could see in his bed. A high fever was the cause of the hallucinations and bacillary dysentery was the cause of the fever. I gave him lots to drink, some acetamino-

Was it supper the night before or the rocking motion of the narrow-gauge railcar? Our two children, aged one and three, started diarrhea as soon as we left Guayaquil. We ran out of diapers and toilet paper. Others were suffering, too—from both ends. The train toilet soon became blocked, but Ecuadorians take such journeys in their stride. Toilet paper was handed round. Jokes flew as everyone shared their resources, and advice. Every time the train broke down, we all used the countryside; seventeen hours later, we chugged into Quito at midnight— parents exhausted but children miraculously recovered.

◆

Jane Vincent-Havelka, over 60, writer/photographer and former traveling mother, London, Ontario, Canada

phen (to lower his high temperature) and sponged him cool. He recovered over the next two days and soon wanted more of those hotel sausages.

The younger a child is, the more they risk serious complications of infectious disease. Infants and toddlers get sicker faster than older children, and may become very unwell indeed if they contract bacillary dysentery. It is also more difficult to identify the source of the problem. Is she unwell, bored, anxious? Parents of small children who travel to less-hygienic countries must read and prepare well before departure; in particular, they must know about oral rehydration therapy and how to recognize dehydration.

Apart from avoiding travelers' diarrhea, the biggest challenge when traveling with children is entertaining them and keeping them happy. The

I'm not a good traveler, and coming back by bus from a sports match, I began to feel really ill. I was carrying my running spikes in a plastic bag and tipped them out and puked into it. Trouble was that the spikes had put holes in the bag and it leaked into my lap.

◆

Alexander Howarth, 13, athlete and cricketer, Ely, UK

most successful project for travelers of any age over about three is to write a "diary." Toward the end of the day, or when waiting around for a bus, get out an exercise book and colored pens and encourage each child to write or draw so that each day they put something on paper. Some will draw whatever they are obsessed with at the time (like castles, airplanes, or dinosaurs), some will draw what they can see, some will record a highlight of the day, like mum slipping in a puddle. Depending upon the age and motivation of the family, you can decorate this with pressed flowers or leaves, or later with photographs. Some parents get the child to dictate what is to be written in the diary while the parent acts as scribe. But the important thing is to get something that the child "owns" down on paper most days of the journey; even a dinosaur drawing will elicit fond memories, and later the child will feel proud of the "book" they have written.

𝒯*ips*

➤ Traveling children must be fully immunized since they are likely to come into contact with unimmunized people and thus their risk of infectious disease is high.

➤ Small children can be scared by dark, unfamiliar toilets (many have no functioning light in less-well-resourced countries), and parents need to go with them. Even during the day, carrying a flashlight will help illuminate the gloom of a basic toilet.

➤ Wise parents travel with toilet paper and also some Wet Wipes.

➤ Children often carry a favorite toy on their visit to the loo; beware that it doesn't fall into the *shaucht*. The latter is an Ulster dialect word for shit.

➤ Families with toddlers who are going to live in the low-income regions should endeavor to find out what kinds of loos are likely to be available. We took a toilet training seat to Nepal only to discover it was useless on our outside squat toilet. Potties, on the other hand, can be useful for older children who wouldn't use them at home; they avoid the need to stroll out into the hazardous mosquito-ridden tropical night.

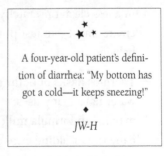

A four-year-old patient's definition of diarrhea: "My bottom has got a cold—it keeps sneezing!"

◆

JW-H

➤ When packing disposable diapers for your child, assume that she will get diarrhea and you will need more diapers than you'd use at home.

➤ Some greasy healing cream will soothe baby's bottom (and his parents') after diarrhea.

➤ Disposable diaper liners make it easier to go for the ecosensitive family option of using cloth diapers rather than disposables, but be aware that even these liners do not compost and are very efficient at blocking up simple flush toilets that are common in the non-industrialized world.

➤ Dispose of soiled diapers sensitively. Bury soiled disposable diapers deep if there is no alternative garbage disposal system. Don't put them in long-drops or composting toilets.

➤ Keep a spare set of clothes in your day bag or flight carry-on bag, in case of unexpected emissions.

➤ Dark-colored underwear is more travel-wise than white.

➤ It is worthwhile keeping a plastic bag in your pocket—traveling children puke a lot.

➤ Changing mats are useful for diaper changes and also—in a less clean or scratchy environment—to just put a baby down.

➤ Thermos flasks of boiling water have many uses: making up formula milk or baby rice, scalding cups and plates, producing safe water, etc. Hot water is especially

In Nepal small children run around with nothing on below the waist. I was painting in a village and, as usual, people gathered around to watch the portrait unfold. Suddenly I felt warm rain falling on my leg: a little boy was peeing while he watched—all over me.

◆

Jan Salter, 61,
British artist, Nepal

invaluable, if the child is at the stage of playfully tossing spoons or cups into the gutter.

➤ Baby pacifiers may be dangerous to small children traveling in unhygienic places. They often fall onto the floor and so become contaminated and then this filth is transferred into the baby's mouth. If the child uses a pacifier, secure it with tape to the child's clothing so that it cannot fall.

➤ True "mineral water" from a natural spring is too high in minerals for small babies to drink safely and should not be used for small infants except in the very short term where there is no alternative. Boiled tap water is safer.

➤ Peel it, boil it, cook it, or forget it, is the mantra to remind you how to keep traveling children free from the squirts in high-risk regions.

As the adolescent male elephant trumpeted, my seven-year-old daughter cringed and I reviewed our situation with carefully concealed rising panic. Was Livingstone (our improbably named guide) faking his cool? Was Kate simply over-reacting? Were we indeed in imminent danger or was the Lariam kicking in? After all, panic attacks were on the list of side effects.

Later Livingstone explained that we'd been "mock charged" by the elephant. Our anxiety had been a very real adrenaline-driven response and not a side effect of the malaria tablets: sometimes though it can be difficult to judge.

◆

Dr. Matthew Ellis, 45, pediatrician and co-author of Your Child Abroad: A Travel Health Guide, *Bristol, UK.*

➤ When traveling in the low-income regions with children, and even on an upmarket beach holiday, it is worth packing a couple of oral rehydration packets.

➤ Beware of buffet food—especially meat dishes—in even the plushest of international hotels.

➤ As with adults, rehydration is important therapy when diarrhea strikes. Any clear fluid will be healing, but mixtures of sugar and salt are absorbed best. If the child will not take ORS (see Chapter 6) then try adding a pinch of salt to a favorite sweet drink like cola.

➤ The first sign of dehydration is a dry lips, and then mouth and tongue.

➤ Seek medical help promptly if in doubt or if the child is becoming too drowsy to drink.

➤ The secret of happy family travel is to have some instant entertainment always on hand in case of delays or queues. I suggest one or two from the following list: small toys such as cars, little figures or plastic animals, balloons, pens and paper, playing cards, favorite storybooks, inflatable beachball, a Frisbee.

We'd planned an eight-day trek with three-month-old Harriet in the middle hills of Nepal, through moderate altitudes along a forested ridge that crossed a road halfway. The first night we reached the misty, damp campsite where it transpired that a (rare) rogue porter had run off with his load including all the disposable diapers. The thief must have been disappointed because our senior porter later found them down a ravine. We set out the next morning thinking nothing else could go wrong, but unseasonal and inauspicious rain clouds clung to our ridge; Harriet was dry under a poncho but she developed a cough. Halfway we decided to hitch back to Kathmandu where Harriet quickly recovered from mild bronchiolitis. Sometimes plans have to change when traveling with children; ensure there is a backup plan, and plenty of diapers.

◆

Dr. Matthew Ellis, 41, pediatrician and co-author of Your Child Abroad, *Bristol, UK*

➤ It can be difficult to know whether a child is really ill or just a little tired or off-color. Taking the child's temperature can often help sort this out: wise parents travel with a thermometer.

➤ When traveling with children under the age of about five years, it is handy to carry some Tylenol (acetaminophen) syrup or chewable tablets from home. Acetaminophen, which is called paracetamol in much of the rest of the world, is widely available but many child formulations are rather unpalatable.

➤ The English are pretty stuffy and unaccommodating of children. If you need to eat out in England, Italian restaurants (or establishments run by southern Europeans) are among the most child-friendly.

We could hardly believe the delights listed on the menu in a tea-house several days from any road in Nepal. They promised pizza, lasagna, chapattis, fresh vegetables as well as the usual rice, lentil slop and vegetable curry. Our boys were excited by the choice and we ordered some of each. We waited a long time and by the time the big shiny metal plates piled with steaming food appeared from the kitchen we were ready to eat anything. It wasn't until we were part way through our tasty meals that we noticed the similarity of all the dishes. Pizza proved to be a chapatti with vegetable curry on top, lasagna was a chapatti and vegetable curry sandwich which didn't look very different from the chapattis and curry.

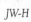

JW-H

Chapter 17

SENIOR TRAVELERS
ASSESSING SPECIAL NEEDS

A sharp-eyed woman who must have been in her eighties described
how she'd flown to Mount Cook in a helicopter. She was a botanical
artist and told the pilot to leave her so she could enjoy absolute
tranquillity. He refused to go at first because if the cloud came down
he would be unable to land again and she'd freeze to death. She
dismissed him anyway. "It is marvelous being old," she said.
"You can be reckless and if you die nobody really minds."

Conversation at a Scientific Exploration Society meeting in London

———

Traveling by rail from Cambridge to London, I fell into conversation with the older gentleman sitting opposite me. He was an architect who'd been involved in designing British Rail facilities. He was disgruntled when he returned from the high-tech loo. "I can't see so well without my glasses, and I wasn't sure what button to press! The designer ought to be shot!"

When I went to investigate I could sympathize. Here is what you do on Great North Eastern Railway trains. Firstly find the button marked <>. It is outside at the level of your belly button. Press to open the big curved door. Then inside just left of the wash basin, find the button >< to close; then press the flashing button with a key symbol on it to lock the door. Then when your organs have been duly evacuated, find the flush button, the water button, the hot air drying button, then the open door button marked <>. If you manage all this you'll be awarded an honorary Ph.D.

Operating the toilet door did seem so unnecessarily complex that I wondered what other challenges travel presents to older travelers or those who have less-than-good eyesight. With aging, it becomes increasingly necessary to prepare properly for any trip, especially if the trip is to be somewhat strenuous. Failing to do this before going trekking can leave you with knees so stiff and painful that you can not use a squat toilet for weeks, and that—in South America or Asia—is disastrous. Even peeing from on high in a squat toilet splatters everything and you need a below-waist shower after every visit.

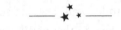

Before I go trekking, I do 100 step-ups on a dining chair; 50 leading with one leg and 50 leading with the other. I do this each day for several days before the trip. This strengthens my thigh muscles to make the first days of the trek less painful, and it also protects my knees from injury.

♦

Jan Salter, 61,
British artist, Nepal

I was up in the mountains in a remote corner of Nepal recently, working in village clinics, sleeping in a single room with my colleagues. Nepali hospitality was pressed upon me daily so by the time we settled to sleep each night I'd be full of tea and middle of the night urinations were inevitable. It is horrible getting up in the night: finding a flashlight but trying not to shine it at anyone, struggling out of a sleeping bag and stepping between sleepers on the floor without disturbing anyone else, unlocking the firmly bolted door then negotiating the route to the outside toilet which always seems to involve clambering over a rickety gate or an unstable dry stone wall. As I've aged and my knees have become more arthritic, squatting has become more challenging. Peeing from a height leaves a big splash-zone and crapping from on high risks missing the target area but only some toilets allow propping up against a wall in order to get down low. Sometimes there's ice on the foot plates. I've concluded that even in the middle of the night and even when it is cold it is best to remove pants and underwear, do the biz, then have a good invigorating splash down. Wearing sandals helps for this bit (but not for negotiating the walls or rough paths). Forgetting the towel is unfortunate. In one toilet in Bajura there was a giant crab spider so large you could hear it as it scuttled across the toilet wall. I wasn't so keen putting out my hand to steady my squat in that particular loo.

Preparations need to include not only physical conditioning but careful packing, too. Have you remembered the contact lens solution, the hormone replacements, and any other regular medicines that you take? A seventy-eight-year-old man consulted me. He was down from the north of England visiting relatives, and he'd forgotten to pack any of the seven different pills he needed to take each day. Worse, he had absolutely no idea what his medicines were, or what they were for. I had to telephone this chap's usual physician before I could prescribe a new set of medicines.

Whatever your age, it is sensible to have a note of any regular medication and keep that note somewhere different from the pills themselves in case your luggage is lost. When traveling abroad, ensure you know the generic name of your medication, since trade names are not international and are rarely intelligible to doctors of other nations who may end up prescribing replacement medicines. By the time the seventy-eight-year-old came to see me his legs were grossly swollen and he was in heart failure, unnecessarily.

Before anyone travels it is important to assess the risks being taken by the particular person in the particular chosen destination. Someone who is taking medicines for heart disease may be more at risk, for example, from electrolyte disturbance in case of diarrhea. Diuretic medicines encourage fluid and electrolyte loss in a way not dissimilar from the fluid and electrolyte loss of diarrhea, and both mechanisms can leave the body depleted of potassium. Blood tests can confirm whether the electrolyte balance is all right, but it may be that you are in a region where reliable laboratory facilities do not exist. Traveling with oral rehydration packets is one obvious precaution, another is being extra cautious about avoiding filth-to-mouth diseases, and even considering whether a trip to a high-risk destination is right for you. If planning a trip to Europe, for example, it will be helpful to know that the risk of diarrheal disease is lower in winter than in summer, and that the risk of the squirts striking in northern Europe is perhaps 8 percent (less than one in ten travelers will suffer in any one trip), whereas for southern Europe it is around 30 percent, one-third.

Five of us celebrated our fiftieth birthdays by different strenuous treks in Nepal; we only discovered this when meeting later. Since then I've trekked in Africa, Irian Jaya, the Himalayas, and the Hindu Kush. A friend celebrated her sixtieth by climbing Kilimanjaro, and I by a month-long pilgrimage to Mt. Kailash, Tibet with a pass at 18,600 feet. I know quite a few over-sixties who have no intention of slowing down yet, but we work at our fitness, and make these challenges a priority in our lives. Mental preparation and stamina are as important as the physical. And we are lucky to have the basic good health which allows us to do this.

◆

Jane Vincent-Havelka, over 60, writer/photographer, London, Ontario, Canada

After someone suffers a blood clot or thrombosis—and this is more common in the over 50s—they are generally instructed to take an anticoagulant (to "thin" the blood) for six months, or sometimes for life. Warfarin is one such anticoagulant. It is an inconvenient medicine as many of the conditions experienced during travel (including changes in diet and illness) can interfere with its efficacy. People taking it also need to have blood tests every two weeks or so and clearly this is not always easy to organize when traveling. Fortunately, newer anticoagulants have been developed which need less stringent monitoring and are little affected by dietary changes. These include edoxaban, apixaban and rivaroxaban. Although these newer anticoagulants are an improvement, all are designed to interfere with the blood's ability to clot and so in case of an accident the result can be disastrous bleeding. Consider the risks therefore and think twice about what might happen after a road accident or other physical trauma and know that medical facilities—and specifically ambulance services—are not uniform the world over, while certain activities and destinations are riskier than others.

Traveling overnight in desert Rajasthan, we did eventually halt briefly in a main street. The public "toilet" consisted of the long wall to the left against which a line of male backs made satisfied Sch-sch-weppes noises, and for me—lone female—the wall to the right where I squatted midway between two streetlights and in imagined privacy relieved my bursting bladder.

◆

Joan Gilchrist, 70, granny
with incurable wanderlust,
Birmingham, UK

With aging the possibility of cancer increases and it is worth knowing that people with cancer have an increased tendency for blood to clot. Cancer treatment may also remove immunity provided by previous immunizations so if planning a big trip to the tropics post-treatment check whether you need to have your childhood and travel immunizations repeated.

Immunization against yellow fever has some special considerations for travelers over the age of 59. The vaccine is now known to provide good life-long protection against the disease (not just for 10 years) but anyone being immunized against yellow fever for the first time after their 60th birthday should be aware that there is an increased chance a serious or even fatal reaction to the vaccine. Discuss your requirements with your physician.

Finally, if you are up in the high mountains and remove your teeth at night, beware. During the misguided invasion of Tibet led by Younghusband in 1903, a British "officer so forgot himself as he bedded down for his first night in Tibet that he put his teeth into a tumbler of water. In the morning he reached for the tumbler and found it frozen solid, his dentures in the midst like a quail in aspic."

Tips

➤ Anyone taking diuretic ("water") tablets or pills to control high blood pressure and who suffers a significant attack of diarrhea should seek medical help promptly if they start to feel dizzy on rising out of a chair or from bed. This is a sign of dehydration (see Chapter 6) and may also indicate the loss of essential electrolytes.

➤ All travelers should know about self-treatment of travelers' diarrhea with oral rehydration solution, and it makes sense to travel with some ORS packets (see page 43).

➤ Those who suffer from diabetes are also likely to become more unwell than nondiabetic travelers when they get diarrhea and should seek a medical consultation if they feel ill. It is all right for diabetics to take ORS (despite the fact it contains glucose). Those whose diabetes is controlled with tablets may temporarily need insulin by injection or via an intravenous drip if the diarrhea is severe.

➤ Anyone who has had a blood clot in the past (or has a close blood relative who has had a clot) is at increased risk of another unless they are taking anticoagulant medicine. The risk also increases with age.

On returning from your holiday, friends invariably ask, "What were the bathrooms like?" There was one in Vietnam with taps to the bath on the opposite side of the bathroom. But the very best places have no bathrooms at all, not even a hole in the ground, until you dig it. Planning your first trip to a wilderness area, the very first thing you must do, especially if you are over fifty, is to take squatting lessons. These can be had at any gymnasium or yoga class. If you don't master prolonged squatting, think again about whether you should risk that trip.

♦

Dr. Jim Waddell, 66, internal medicine physician, Cirencester, UK

➤ Some ongoing medical conditions make long-haul trips or travel to very remote regions unwise. Ask your doctor what is sensible. Bad backs, for example, are made more painful by long car journeys and probably also by long jarring bus rides.

➤ Take plenty of any medicines that you need and preferably pack them in two different bags in case an item of luggage is lost or delayed. Also travel with a list of all medicines you take, their generic names, and the exact doses. Never assume that you will be able to replenish your tablets at your destination.

➤ When planning a long, intercontinental journey that you expect to be tiring or stressful, consider buying a business-class ticket. This costs more but provides a comfortable, uncrowded waiting area before boarding, and much more space and more attentive service in flight. You thus arrive fresher and are less likely to feel that you need to recover before starting to enjoy your travel experience.

➤ If business-class travel is not feasible, ensure—at least— that your flight times are convenient. Many cut-priced tickets have you flying on unpleasant, sleep-depriving schedules.

➤ Anyone who can walk fifty yards without becoming breathless should be able to tolerate the reduced oxygen in flight. Check with your doctor if you want to know if you are fit to fly.

➤ Research any stop-overs if you dislike walking far. Some airports, Frankfurt for example, are huge.

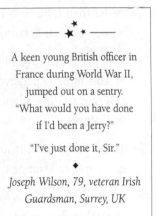

A keen young British officer in France during World War II, jumped out on a sentry. "What would you have done if I'd been a Jerry?"

"I've just done it, Sir."

◆

Joseph Wilson, 79, veteran Irish Guardsman, Surrey, UK

➤ Bring along an extra pair of eyeglasses or a copy of your eyeglass prescription; replacements bought in the low-income regions can be remarkably inexpensive.

➤ Those who have difficulty squatting should do some quadriceps strengthening exercises before travel. Women might like to buy a Shewee (see page 116) or one of several washable devices that allow women to pee standing up.

➤ If some illness strikes just before your planned trip, give serious thought to whether it would be better to postpone the trip. It is no fun traveling ill, and doctors at your destination are likely to have very different, unfamiliar consultation styles, which may not be very reassuring.

➤ Try to make a hard, rational assessment of your capabilities before any trip and make sure you are up to it. Get fit for your trip because aging bodies need more training for unfamiliar activities. I have met many trekkers, more than twenty years my senior, yet managing the physical demands better than I, but it is clear that these travelers have invested a lot of time in keeping in condition.

➤ People over the age of seventy-five may find it difficult (or at least more expensive) to rent a car or arrange travel insurance. Allow plenty of time for such arrangements; plan well ahead.

➤ Travel with health insurance—even if this is difficult or expensive to arrange.

➤ Cruise ships and long-distance tour buses are great places to catch airborne rotaviruses, Norovirus, or Norwalk-like viruses. These cause epidemic vomiting; the incubation interval is 15 to 50 hours and symptoms settle in 48 hours.

In Ashgabat, Turkmenistan, I craved privacy. I searched to no avail, then located a guard and somehow made him understand my urgent need. I walked up and down and outside and on and on, my legs no longer straight and underwear hot and sweaty, to a place in the middle of rickety buildings where an old half-unhinged door radiated an unmistakable smell. How I got into it and squatted down without touching anything is another story. Paper there was none, but an old Kleenex in my bag did the job. After getting out as fast as I could the smell still harassed me for a long while.

◆

Françoise Hivernel, 66, archaeologist, psychoanalyst author of Safartu *and contributor to* 50 Camels *and* She's Yours, *Waterbeach, UK*

Chapter 18

HOMECOMING
YOU'VE RETURNED, ARE YOU HEALTHY?

Simagaul arrived with his *charriot-aux-boeufs* for the last time. He
asked for a third course of antibiotics for STIs, but I was unsure
whether he had actually got it again or only intended to.... We
loaded the cart with rucksacks and made our final walk through the
forest of the Canyon Grande. Armand guided us out across the
savannah to a junction of two dirt tracks, about eight miles from
camp, where a bush taxi passed at 11 A.M. each day. He picked
some custard apples and ate them with us before he departed. It
had been a good expedition. I sat in the shade, so sad to be leaving,
but musing greedily on the culinary delights awaiting us in Diégo-
Suarez. It would not take me long to replace the fifteen pounds of
fat I had lost during my two and a half months in Madagascar.

—Jane Wilson, *Lemurs of the Lost World*

───────

The vast majority of travelers return from their exotic
adventures feeling very well, yet they often have concerns about tropical hitchhikers. Feeling well does not
necessarily dispel the thought that some weird infection might
be lurking within, soon to break out and overwhelm them. Is
this likely? The answer is "no." Fortunately, almost all tropical
diseases and infections will cause some kind of symptoms so
that you can take yourself to the doctor for treatment. And
those that don't cause symptoms rarely need treatment. There
are, of course, a few exceptions and it is worth mentioning
those to be aware of.

Perhaps the most common health problem, especially after
returning from a long, perhaps life-changing trip, is connected
with mood. It can be quite an anticlimax coming back,

realizing that life has gone on perfectly well without you. You may need to find a job, somewhere to live; you may find it hard initially to find kindred spirits to talk to. Depression can creep up on you. Be aware that "post-trip blues" are common, and the best treatment is to link up with other returned travelers and talk about your feelings. And if your moods are unbearably low much of the time, you are not sleeping well, or you are tearful, seek medical help. Usually it is a passing phenomenon and you'll get back to normal, only richer for the experience.

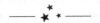

Happy memories. Memories of China and the holes in the floor which are the only toilets in the world I have ever seen maggots trying to get out of. Memories of India, and men by the road-side peeing behind the huge and wonderful Bollywood billboards that only come down to chest height so that everything below was on view to road-users.

◆

Tim Burford, 46, author for Bradt Travel Guides and the Rough Guides, Cambridge, UK

Malaria can catch travelers unaware so that they become rapidly ill. Sub-Saharan Africa is a common place to contract malaria, whether or not you have taken precautions against the disease. Realize when and where you might risk malaria. Symptoms begin at least a week after the first bite and usually within three months of return, but possibly up to a year of leaving a malarious region. Seek medical help urgently if you become feverish with aches and pains, and you think you could have malaria.

Did you put yourself at risk of HIV on your travels? Symptoms are rare initially but a screening blood test will tell you whether you have become infected. And similarly bilharzia, the disease acquired from paddling or swimming in infected freshwater in Africa and parts of tropical South America (see pages 123–126), may cause no symptoms but a blood test done more than six weeks from your last possible exposure will tell you if you need treatment.

Apart from those exceptions, almost all other infections will cause telltale symptoms. Those who have been traveling independently in countries with poor sanitation often pick up a worm or two, but in small numbers they are most unlikely to harm you. Probably the first you will know of their presence is passing one once it comes to the end of its life (see Chapter 12).

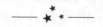

You know what was nice about Cartegena—toilet seats. Nowhere else that I stayed in Colombia had them. We take a lot of things for granted but it's not until you wee out four bottles of *cerveza* while sitting with your balls dangling low to the rising tide in the toilet bowl that you reflect on the important things in life.

◆

Calvin Dorion, 35, teacher, Cambridge, UK

It doesn't matter whether you get these treated or not, but if you are squeamish about the possibility of carrying worms, organize a stool test.

Tips

➢ Remember the risk of serious malaria and seek medical help urgently (within twenty-four hours) if you fall ill within three months of returning from the tropics—even if you have taken your antimalarial tablets.

➢ Malaria can make you ill any time from one week to up to a year after exposure to malarious mosquitoes. Help your physician by reminding him where you have been.

➢ With the exception of Malarone, antimalarial tablets should be continued for four weeks after returning from your travels; they are not an absolute guarantee that you will avoid malaria, but if you are unlucky enough to get it, you are less likely to die of it.

➤ Other diseases imported from the tropics are unlikely to be serious, but seek a medical opinion if you notice a rash, an ulcer that refuses to heal, new lumps or bumps, or are unwell. Remind your doctor that you have been abroad.

➤ If you are feeling down after your trip, find a kindred spirit to talk to.

➤ Do not worry about your health on your return; if you feel well, you almost certainly are well.

As global citizens, we can curb our impact on the natural world, as well as staying safe ourselves, by considering our mode of transport and our diets.

Travel slowly rather than jetting around and it may surprise you with just how easy it is to save precious carbon. You might even find yourself relaxing, saving money, and experiencing something that you couldn't have dreamed of.

One of the best aspects of travel is experiencing new culinary delights, but we can still sample a culture while remaining cognizant of where this food came from. Eating more plant-based foods will dramatically decrease your ecological footprint and the exploitation of wild places that we love to visit as well as cut the diarrhea risk.

◆

Sebastian Howarth, 25, research fellow at Utopia, Kathmandu, Nepal

Chapter 19

PACKING LIST AND
MINIMAL MEDICAL KIT

——

M y first big trip to the tropics was when I was 22 and I set out weighed down with a ridiculous quantity of medicaments, most of which I gave away. Now I am older and wiser and these days when I travel I take very little. My recommended absolute minimum first-aid kit is:

➤ A good drying antiseptic (e.g., iodine or potassium permanganate)—don't take antiseptic cream. Remember skin infections are common in the tropics

➤ A few small dressings (Band-Aids plus some larger nonstick dressings and micropore tape to stick them on with). Scrapes and grazes need covering against flies and other insects

➤ Steristrips—tape for pulling the edges of large wounds together

➤ Insect repellent; malaria tablets; impregnated mosquito net

➤ Condoms (they also can be useful emergency water carriers)

➤ Sunscreen with a protection factor (SPF) of 15 or more

➤ Acetaminophen (paracetamol) or ibuprofen—soluble forms are good for gargling to soothe a sore throat

➤ Antifungal cream (e.g., Daktarin or Canesten) for athlete's foot and groin itches

➤ Greasy soothing cream or hemorrhoid treatment for the overexerted anus

➤ An antibiotic in case of severe diarrhea: xifaxan/rifaximin/xifaxanta 200mg x9 or azithromycin 500mg x 2

➤ Another broad-spectrum antibiotic like amoxicillin or (if penicillin allergic) erythromycin (for chest, urine, skin infections, etc.)

➤ A pair of fine pointed tweezers for removing thorns, coral fragments, caterpillar hairs, etc.

➤ Nail clippers or scissors

Here are few more hygiene-related items that you might need when traveling in regions with poor infrastructure:'

➤ Reliable flashlight (preferably a headlight)

➤ Toilet paper

➤ Wet wipes

➤ Disposable cleaning cloths or a washcloth

➤ Large dark-colored (green, navy) bath towel and maybe a sarong

➤ Resealable plastic bags or at least a few plastic shopping bags (for vomit or soiled clothes)

➤ One or two good quality one-liter water bottles

➤ Iodine to purify the water (and also useful when diluted as an antiseptic) and vitamin C to improve the taste, or a water purification device

➤ Vacuum flask—especially valuable when traveling with
   small children

➤ Oral rehydration packets—check that the cup or bottle that
   you carry is the correct volume for making up ORS

➤ A few Oxo stock (boullion) cubes for making savory drinks
   during diarrhea

➤ An oral rehydration "recipe" (see page 44)

➤ Plastic containers to mix rehydration solutions and carry
   liquids

➤ A fine-toothed comb (for lice) especially if traveling with
   children

➤ Women's sanitary items sealed in good waterproof container
   or plastic bags

➤ A list of any medicines you take with a note of their
   generic names

➤ Spare eyeglasses or eyeglasses prescription

➤ Immunization certificates

➤ At least one good, long novel.

References

Arscott, David. *Sussex Privies: A Nostalgic Trip Down the Garden Path.* Newbury Berkshire, UK: Countryside Books, 1998.

At Your Convenience: Public Toilets Around the World. London: Ebury Press, 2001.

Belamy, David. *Poo You and the Potoroo's Loo.* London: Portland Press, 1997. Neat children's book about environmental responsibilities.

Bezruchka, Stephen, M.D. *Altitude Illness: Prevention and Treatment.* Seattle: The Mountaineers, 2005. A helpful, accessible guide; essential reading for trekkers.

Bezruchka, Stephen, M.D. *The Pocket Doctor: A Passport to Healthy Travel (3rd ed.).* Seattle: The Mountaineers, 1999. Covers preparations, precautions, and care while abroad. A sensible, helpful guide in a conveniently small format.

Centers for Disease Control. *Health Information for International Travel 2005-2006.* Atlanta, GA: CDC, 2005. Best English-language publication for international disease risks information, though hardly an entertaining read. Updated every two years. Single copies are available from CDC (Attention Health Information), Center for Prevention Services, Division of Quarantine, Atlanta, GA 30333, USA.

Cho, Shinta, and Amanda Mayer Stinchecum. *The Gas We Pass: The Story of Farts.* La Jolla, CA: Kane / Miller Book Publishers, 2001; for children.

Gomi, Taro, and Amanda Mayer Stinchecum. *Everyone Poops.* La Jolla, CA: Kane / Miller Book Publishers, 2001; for children.

Johnson, Chris, Sarah Anderson, Warrell, David, et al (eds.). *Oxford Handbook of Expedition and Wilderness Medicine.* Oxford: Oxford University Press, 2020. All you need to know about health and illness on expeditions including how to build a latrine. Written by senior expedition physicians. Warrell is professor at the Oxford University Medical School and a world authority on venomous creatures.

Lewin, Ralph A. *Merde: Excursions into Scientific, Cultural and Socio-Historical Coprology.* New York: Random House, 1999.

Meyer, Kathleen. *How to Shit in the Woods.* Berkeley, CA: Ten Speed Press, 1994. Practical advice for backcountry travel as well as environmental methods for keeping wild places pristine, aesthetically and bacterially. www.KathleenintheWoods.net

Newman, Eva. *Going Abroad: The Bathroom Survival Guide.* St. Paul, MN: Marlor Press, 2000. A guide to unfamiliar toilets.

Reyburn, Wallace. *Flushed with Pride: The Story of Thomas Crapper.* London: Pavilion Books, 1989.

Turner, Jean. *East Anglian Privies: A Nostalgic Trip Down the Garden Path.* Newbury Berkshire, UK: Countryside Books, 1998.

Van der Ryn, Sim. *The Toilet Papers: Recycling Waste and Conserving Water.* London: Chelsea Green Publishing, 1999.

Where to GO in the Great Outdoors. Mountaineering Council of Scotland. 4A St Catherine's Rd, Perth PH1 5SE (send SAE). Phone 01738-638229, fax 01738-442095. Useful pamphlet for walkers in Britain.

Wilson-Howarth, Jane. *Staying Healthy When You Travel: avoiding bugs bites bellyaches and more.* Mount Joy, PA, US: Fox Chapel Publishing, 2020. Accessible health information written by a physician who has practiced in low income countries for 14 years and in the UK for even longer. Comprehensive and contains instructive case histories to learn from.

Wilson-Howarth, Jane, and Matthew Ellis. *Your Child Abroad: a travel health guide.* Chalfont St. Peter, UK: Bradt Travel Guides, 2014. Written by two physicians who are also widely-travelled parents.

World Health Organization. *International Travel and Health.* Geneva, Switzerland: World Health Organization Publications, 2005. Annually updated booklet; dry reading.

NEWSLETTERS AND JOURNALS

www.lonelyplanet.com/magazine/
Rough guides travel news www.roughguides.com/article/travel-news-round-up/

Wanderlust magazine comes out 10 times a year and each issue carries a feature on some aspect of travel health. There is also a newsletter https://www.wanderlust.co.uk

World Nomads www.worldnomads.com produce entertaining and informative podcasts on travel

SERVICES AND ORGANIZATIONS

Canadian Department of Trade and Foreign Affairs official one stop travel shop www.travel.gc.ca

Centers for Disease Control (CDC)
Atlanta, Georgia 30333 USA
Website: www.cdc.gov
The CDC is the central source of travel health information in North America. They publish each summer the invaluable *Health Information for International Travel*.

International Association for Medical Assistance to Travellers (IAMAT)
1623 Military Rd. #279 Niagara Falls, NY 14304-1745
Phone 716 754 4883
https://www.iamat.org
A nonprofit foundation that provides lists of English-speaking doctors abroad as well as foreign health information.

INTERNET RESOURCES

Centers for Disease Control and Prevention
www.cdc.gov/travel/
Includes a country by country list of immunizations and advice on malaria risk, www.cdc.gov/travel

Fit for Travel
www.fitfortravel.nhs.uk
This comprehensive website by the National Health Service in Scotland presents information on specific travel destinations, with guidelines for special groups such as children, pregnant travelers, and elderly travelers.

International Association for Medical Assistance
to Travellers (IAMAT)
www.iamat.org
Advises travelers of health risks, geographical distribution of
diseases, immunization requirements, as well as providing lists
of English-speaking doctors throughout the world.

International Society of Travel Medicine
www.istm.org
The big organization for health professionals. Provides a search
facility to help you find a travel clinic anywhere in the world.

ProMED
www.promedmail.org
and the International Society for Infectious Diseases
A global electronic reporting system for outbreaks of emerging
infectious diseases. Contains current alerts (outbreaks in animals are even included), disease outbreak maps, and articles on
travel health. Available in English, Portuguese, Spanish,
Chinese, and Japanese.

Travel Health Online
www.tripprep.com
This website provides health and safety information on more than
220 countries, including immunization recommendations, preven-
tions, warnings, travel medical providers, and health concerns.

www.trexmed.co.uk/schistosomiasis-bilharzia
for an accessible expert view on schistosomiasis aka bilharzia

World Health Organization
www.who.int/en

And just for fun thebathroomdiaries.com

INDEX

———

INDEX OF CONTRIBUTORS

Acknowledgments

———

This little book started with a germ of an idea of Sean O'Reilly's, and he called me in Kathmandu to ask me to write about shitting abroad. This unusual request was the start of an enjoyable transatlantic email relationship with the editors and staff of Travelers' Tales. Thanks to Susan Brady, Larry Habegger, and James O'Reilly who have come up with excellent suggestions. Most outside contributions came in response to a plea in *Wanderlust*, the British travel magazine for whom I write regularly (thanks to editor, Lyn Hughes) but I also received material from members of the Scientific Exploration Society of Great Britain; thank you to Wendy Bentall, editor of the SES newsletter *Sesame*. Friends, relations, acquaintances, and other members of the International Society of Travel Medicine have directed me toward unexpected sources and helped improve the information within these pages. I especially want to mention contributions from Ann Bevan, Hilary Bradt, Sarah Geeson-Brown, and Susanna Maybin. Sadly since the last edition of this book was published three of our contributors, Jan Salter, Jean Sinclair and Greg Whiteside, have passed on from this world too soon but I am proud that their wisdom is still being shared.

I am also enormously grateful to my husband Simon Howarth for being his usual quiet supportive self. Many of the tales within these pages were collected whilst we've traveled together over the past years. I also appreciate my parents' liberal views in tolerating a daughter who talks crap and writes filth.

About the Author

Dr. Jane Wilson-Howarth achieved a pinnacle of professional development by being invited to teach on diarrhea at Cambridge University Medical School. The path that has led to that dubious distinction started with a childhood interest in creepy-crawlies which drove her to study zoology and then organize a six-month-long expedition to the Himalayas to research lesser wildlife there. Interested in cave life, she soon discovered that a lot could be learned from the brown deposits animals leave behind, as well as from watching creatures themselves. She spent a couple of years at Oxford University studying rabbit parasites, then entered medical school where her friends called her the Shit Doctor because of a continuing interest in parasites and poo. On completion of her studies, she was awarded a BM—a bachelor of medicine degree; this is equivalent to the American MD qualification.

She organized two research trips to Madagascar where dunes of bat guano hid rare species of invertebrates unknown to science. She also watched and photographed attractive creatures, completing the first ever study of the endangered Crowned Lemur in the wild; this involved meticulous observations, and—of course—examinations of their emanations. Her first book, *Lemurs of the Lost World*, describes the Madagascar expeditions. Field studies in Peru continued on the ecology of excreta and she worked where mounds of subterranean guano seethed with fascinating crawlies, and where spelunkers risked catching histoplasmosis and rabies. She has discovered and documented an array of dung-eating invertebrates that were unknown to science.

She has lived in Asia for fourteen years, working on child survival and preventing diarrheal disease in Sri Lanka, Indonesia, Pakistan, India, Bangladesh, and Nepal mostly in communities lacking reliable power supplies, sewage arrangements, or paved road access. Some of this work involved screening people for worms and also encouraging villagers to build and use latrines. Her experiences in Nepal are described in her second memoir, *A Glimpse of Eternal Snows*. She has also written four novels set in Nepal, one for adults and three for children.

These days, she divides her time between Cambridge UK and Kathmandu and teaches, writes and lectures including on travel and health. She especially enjoys giving pre-departure briefings to VSO volunteers as well as to relief and humanitarian workers–giving them a toolkit to ensure they stay healthy on their missions. Her UK home boasts three flushing sit-down loos. Her two comprehensive travel heath guides are *Your Child Abroad: a travel health guide* (Bradt Travel Guides) and *Staying Healthy While You Travel: avoiding bugs bites bellyaches and more* (Fox Chapel Publishing). Her author website is www.wilson-howarth.com, she tweets (occasionally) as @longdropdoc and her Instagram account is also @longdropdoc.